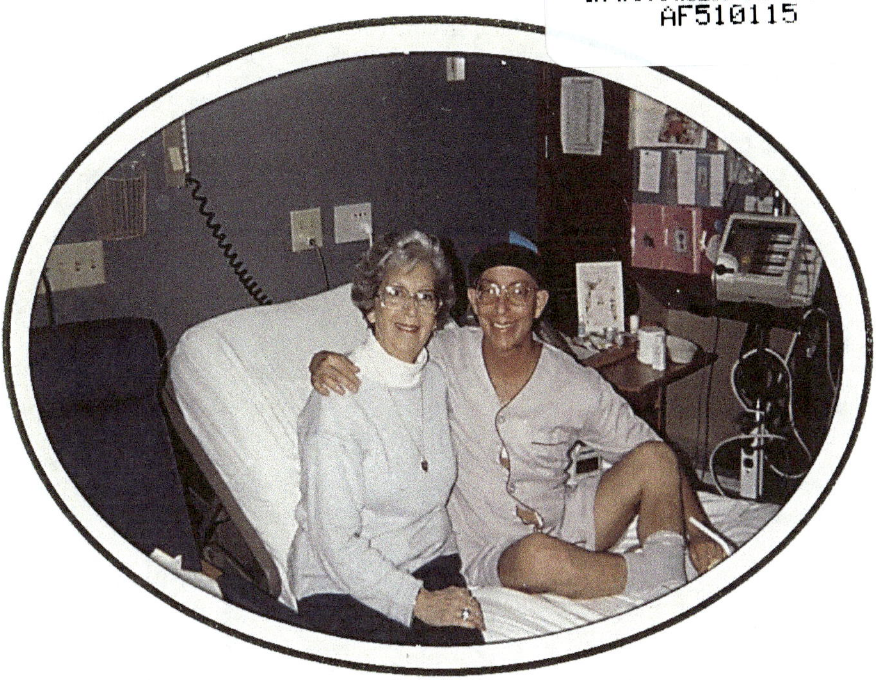

One Life To Live

My Journey Through Health, Healing, And Faith
-Surviving Stage 4 Cancer

By

Barton H. Dunn

Introduction

I remember when I was only five years old, I walked to the end of the driveway; I looked up to the sky and asked God to watch over me. I knew that somehow, I was different and just asked for guidance in my life. I truly believe that God hears all of our prayers. In this book, you will read about the many trials and tribulations in my life like having stage 4 A.L.L Leukemia, three times with Shekinah glory. God is real. God is still with us, and God continues to perform miracles! And I am one of them!

Prologue

As you read my story, you will find out about my background growing up to walking into my Doctor's office thinking I had the flu. Three days later, I woke up in the intensive care unit at the Hospital with stage 4 A.L.L leukemia (Cancer of the blood). To God making me a Prophet to help a family in grief, too telling my story every single day for the rest of my life. I am writing this book to get my story out to more people.

I hope you are inspired by my story and, as Paul Harvey would say, "And now the rest of the story."

IHS

Bart H. Dunn

Dedicated to God and Steve Dunn (My Twin Brother) the Dunn Family, and Dennis Cantile

Table Of Contents

Chapter 1
Childhood

Now, a little bit about me and who I am.

Describe my childhood in 3 words:

Blessed, Interesting, Enjoyable

I was born on 3/31/1957 at Albert Einstein Hospital in Philly, Pa. My identical twin brother Steve was born 1 minute before me. We were born premature 3 ½ months. Steve weighted 3 lbs and I weighted 2 ½ lbs. To survive this was a miracle in 1957. We lived in Philadelphia, PA, for two years in a row house. I don't remember much at that age. We then moved down to Charlotte, NC. My Mom & Dad, my twin Steve, my middle brother Gary, and my oldest brother Lance made the move in 1959. At two years old, moving to Charlotte, NC, was a big change for us.

We moved to a single-story wood house on Vale Ave. off of Randolph Road for about 9 months. We later moved to Lynbrook Dr. My Dad had built our 2nd house built of brick Gray/white house out towards Rama Road and Sardis Road).

The city limits were at Rama Road back in 1960. We built our 2nd house living in Charlotte on Lynbrook Drive, and farmland all the way to Monroe, NC. There was one traffic light from Charlotte to Monroe, NC which is a 30-mile drive.

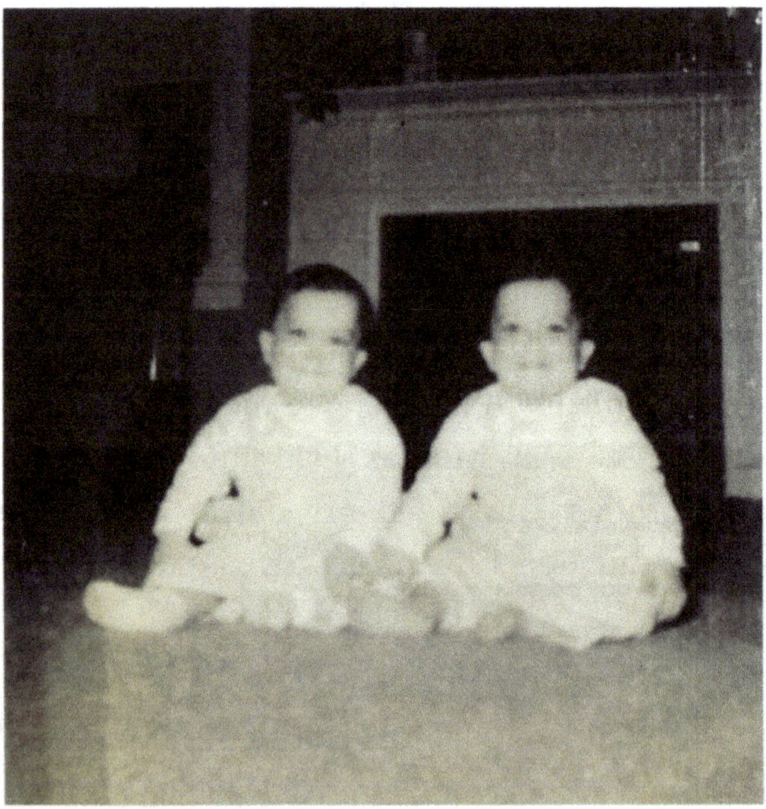

Bart and Steve 1 year old

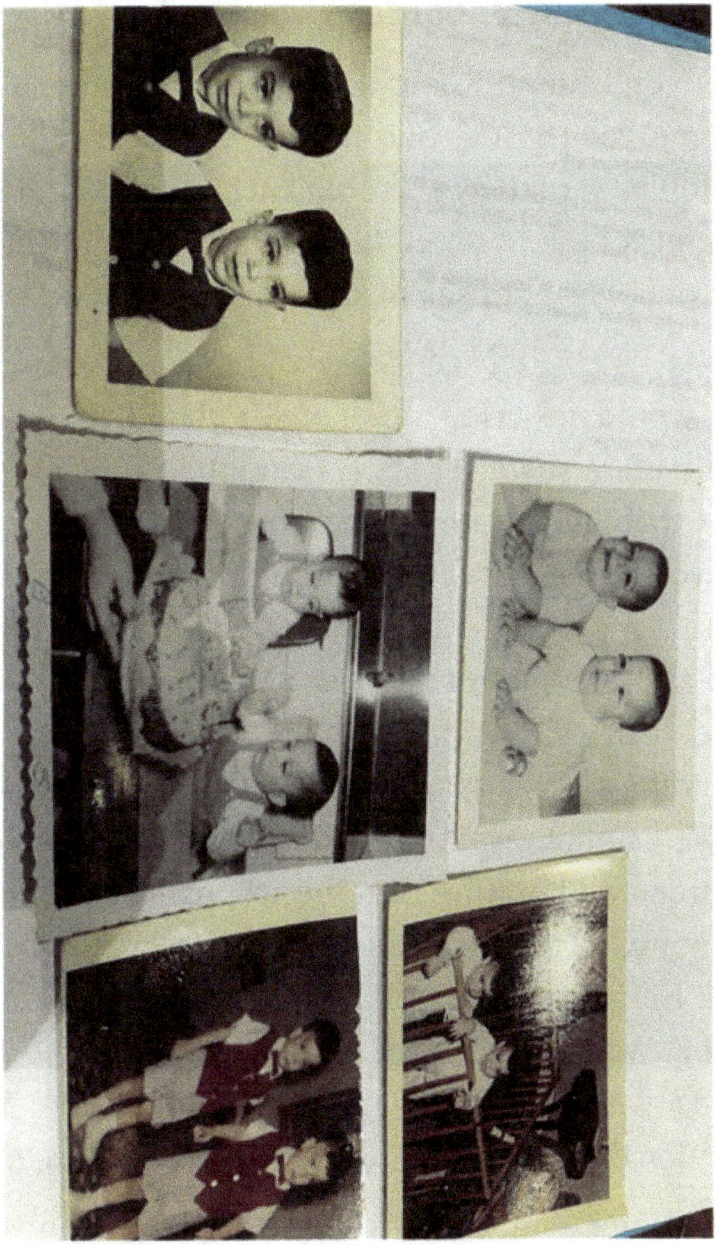

Bart and Steve one to three years old

Describe the neighborhood you grew up in:

Beyond Rama Road, it was all farmland and trees. We enjoyed living out in the country before the development of the widespread neighborhood. Most of the homes on our street were built in the 1960s. Most were one-story houses made of brick, and some were wood. Most of the lots were 1 acre with trees.

I would describe our neighborhood as a upper-middle class section of S.E Charlotte. The streets are wide with many types of trees, like Elm, Poplar, Dogwood, Pine, Redbud, and many more. I like the fact that most of the homes were built in the 60s, the front and back yards are very large, plenty of space between them. By the 70s, the neighborhoods were expanding outwards at Rama Road and Sardis Road. We were able to walk to our Elementary school, down the street, and cutting thru the woods. We would ride the swings at the playground. Then, walk up the field to the Elementary school. This was about 1 /2 miles to school, which was very convenient. We had many friends who lived in our neighborhood. We had a neighbor Burnett who lived behind our house.

Burnette's mother Dottie lost her first husband, Ralph in the early 1960s, and then she married Bob in

1964. He was a building contractor and built South Park Mall, which opened on Feb 12, 1970. It was located on Sharon Road and the corner of Fair View Road. The South Park area in South Charlotte was once a thriving 3,000-acre dairy farm owned by NC Governor Cameron Morrison.

Chapter 2
Famous Bus Ride

An adventure trip from our house by bus around Charlotte, NC, which was a 3-hour tour almost like Gilligan's Island. At the time, we were 4 years old. But our trip was so much better. The date was July 13, 1961 Thursday. I decided on that early morning to do something fun and exciting that we both would enjoy. It's hard to believe that I thought of this trip at that age. I guess we wanted to do something really different from our normal activities.

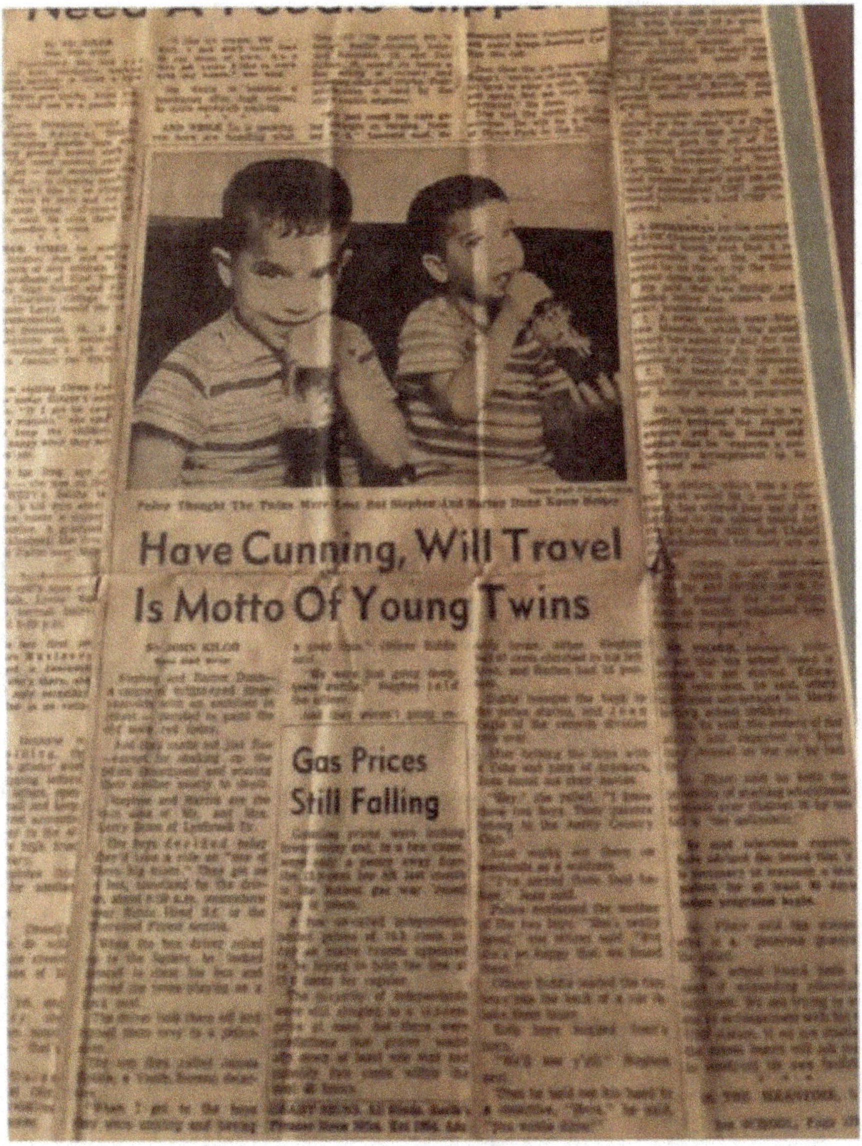

Have Cunning, Will Travel Is Motto Of Young Twins

Gas Prices Still Falling

3 hour tour of Charlotte, NC 1961

Steve had sixty-seven cents, and I had just fifteen pennies clinched in my hand ready to leave our house for an adventure. We walked out the side door so as not to wake up our mother. We walked out toward the end of the driveway and turned right, down the street up the hill, and made a left at the Stop sign which was Doncaster Street. We walked for 30 minutes and turned right up the hill to the Bus stop at Nottingham St. There were approximately Twelve maids waiting to be picked up by the city bus.

As the bus approached and stopped, several maids hopped on the bus. When the last maid got onto the bus, we hopped on too and passed the meter change box.

The driver did not question us since he thought we were with the last maids that got onto the bus. We went to the back of the bus and sat in the backseat in the middle.

As we approached each bus stop, one or more maids would exit the bus. One hour turned into 3 hours as the rest of the maids hopped off the last bus stop. By now, the bus driver noticed us playing in the backseat alone while the bus was empty except for us two!

The bus driver yelled toward the back of the bus, “Why did You not get off with one of the maids?”

Steve then said, “They don't belong to us.” The frantic driver ran down the center aisle and said to us, “We are getting off here at Trade and Tryon Street,” and then we walked 10 minutes to the police station! When we arrived at the station, we were given to James Biddle, a youth bureau detective. When he came into the room, we were smiling and having a good time: “We were just going downtown for a while,” Steve told the officer.

Biddle brought the boys to Joan (Officer Biddle’s assistant). After bribing the boys with a glass Bottle of Coke and a pack of Lance Crackers, “HEY!” she yelled. “I know these two boys! Their parents belong to the Amity Country Club”. Joan works out there on weekends as a waitress. “I've served them food before.” She has waited on our family for several years, Joan said.

The Police contacted our mother. “She is really upset”, the officer said. “But so glad they were found ok.” Officer Biddle loaded us into the back of the police car to take us back home now that he had our address.

We hugged Joan’s neck and said goodbye. “We’ll see y’all”, Steve said. Then he held out his hand to the detective, "Here," he said, "You wanna dime!". We couldn't wait to tell Mom that Joan worked at the police station. We arrived back home and Mom was still very upset. Mom said, "Why did you leave the house?" I said, "I am the one who talked Steve into going on our trip." "I'm very sorry for doing that." (we still got a spanking from Dad when he came home.)

This was such a fantastic story. We were on the Front-Page of the paper (Charlotte Observer), on TV, and on the radio. No one in the Charlotte area had ever seen something like this before.

The Charlotte Newspaper had a front headline, "Have cunning, Will Travel, is the Motto of young twins."

This event Will be remembered for a very long time. By the way, at that time the price of gas was only 16 cents per gallon.

In 2011, Fifty years after the first bus ride downtown, The Charlotte Observer did a follow-up story that reminds me of how fast time flies by. I remember the journey as if it were yesterday. Most of the residents of Charlotte still remember that special day that took the city by surprise. What would you think if this event happened now? Would it be such a shock story today if young twins took a 3-hour bus ride around Charlotte in 2024? I believe it would still be a shock factor if it happened today! I remember this classic bus ride my twin brother Steve and I took just for the fun of it. As the Comedian Bob Hope would say, "Thanks for the Memories."

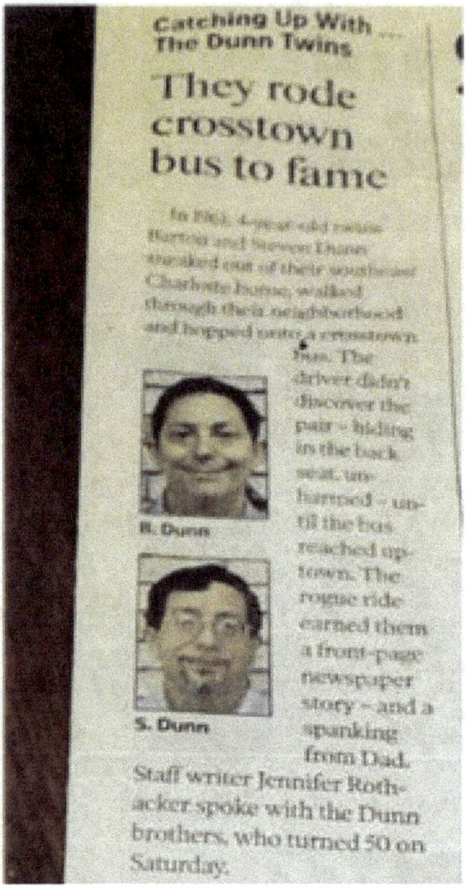

Catching Up With ... The Dunn Twins

They rode crosstown bus to fame

In [illegible], [illegible]-year-old twins Barton and Steven Dunn sneaked out of their southeast Charlotte home, walked through their neighborhood and hopped onto a crosstown bus. The driver didn't discover the pair – hiding in the back seat, unharmed – until the bus reached uptown. The rogue ride earned them a front-page newspaper story – and a spanking from Dad.

B. Dunn

S. Dunn

Staff writer Jennifer Rothacker spoke with the Dunn brothers, who turned 50 on Saturday.

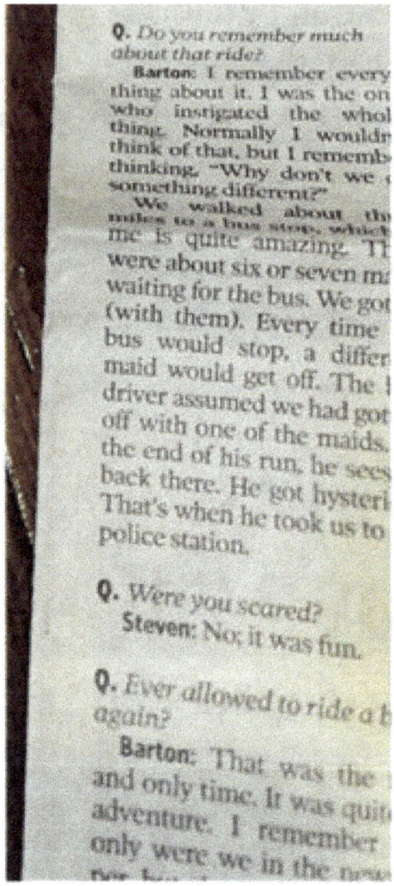

Q. *Do you remember much about that ride?*

Barton: I remember every thing about it. I was the on who instigated the whol thing. Normally I wouldn think of that, but I rememb thinking, "Why don't we something different?"

We walked about th [illegible] me is quite amazing. Th were about six or seven ma waiting for the bus. We got (with them). Every time bus would stop, a differ maid would get off. The driver assumed we had got off with one of the maids. the end of his run, he sees back there. He got hysteri That's when he took us to police station.

Q. *Were you scared?*

Steven: No, it was fun.

Q. *Ever allowed to ride a b again?*

Barton: That was the and only time. It was quit adventure. I remember only were we in the new

Follow up story from Bus Ride Charlotte, NC

Schooling

I went to East Mecklenburg High School in Charlotte, NC. After graduation from High School, I decided to go to onward College (in 1975).

Mars Hill College 1975-1979, University of Tampa 1979-1980

What did you love most about school?

Both this college and university were small private schools. I liked that the classes were small in number, and you were able to see friends more often around campus. I believe the professors were able to give more attention to the students. I really enjoyed meeting people from around the country who later became friends. I graduated in 1980 from the University of Tampa with a BS Degree in Business Management and Economics. My parents came to Tampa for my graduation. I enjoyed the warmer temperatures in Tampa. l really enjoyed my classes. I enjoyed the field trips we took from my business class. I am so glad I went to college. I wish to say how grateful I am that my parents made that opportunity possible for me and my three brothers (Lance, Gary and Stove).

Anything else you'd like to add about your schooling years?

I went to college from 1975-1980. These were some of the best times in my life. In 1977 (my sophomore year at college), My twin brother Steve and I took a 5-week backpacking trip/Railroad trip from London England down to Algiers, Morocco. This was the most exciting trip I have ever had at that time of my life. I have been to many destination places and cruises Too many to count!

What did you dislike most about school?

At Mars Hill College, which is located about 20 miles North of Asheville, NC, The only dislike I had about this school was it was very cold in the winter months, sometimes 2 feet of snow, and walking down all the steps from Gibson Hall. This was the nice dorm and the most modern dorm.

I had no dislikes from the University of Tampa

Do you remember any fads from school?

I went to Mars Hill College during the Disco Era.

Which "group" were you in?

I did belong to the Hiking Club and the History Club at Mars Hill College. I had a very diverse group of friends.

What did you do for fun?

I started collecting coins in the 9th grade. This is a hobby that I have had all my life. I like to collect silver and gold coins and paper money. I also like to go Gem Mining up toward the mountains of North Carolina. I like taking day trips around NC. I enjoy going to antique shops.

Who was your best friend in school, and how did you meet them?

I lived in Charlotte, NC, South East, off of Rama Road on Lynbrook Drive. My best friend was Burnett, who lived behind us on Riviera Drive. My other best friend was Andrew, who lived on Riviera Drive, too. These two friends lived very close so it was easy to hang out together! My Elementary school, Junior, and High school were only within 5 miles between one and the other two.

It was great having so many friends living so close together. Other close friends are Mark, we have been friends for 61 years. We met in the first grade. Jeff and I have been friends for 54 years. All of our birthdays are close together.

In school, what did you want to be when you grew up?

Before going off to College, I knew I wanted to study Business and Economics. My goal was to study and graduate from college.

This was a prerequisite before going into the family Textile Business. I have been working in the Family business from 1980 to the present.

My first college choice was Mars Hill College, Mars Hill, NC. This college is located about 20 miles north of Asheville, NC. I wanted to attend a college close to home which is Charlotte, NC. The drive is approx. 3 hours door to door. This allowed me to drive home to visit Mom and Dad on the weekends.

I studied Business and Economics in my 5th year at the Univ. of Tampa, Tampa, FI.

Chapter 3
Work

Which word do you most associate with your work?

Devoted

Describe a typical day in your job.

I have been working in sales for most of the 43 years working at Dunn Trimming and Binding. In 2008, I was promoted to Vice President of the company. Customers send in fabric, and we biased the fabric on a 45% angle, re-roll the fabric and cut it in different sizes (ie:1"bias, 2"bias, etc.). We also have straight-cut fabric and crosscut, which means you don't have any seams.

We have broadcloth fabric in 100 colors and offer other fabrics available. Our website is www.dunntrimming.com. In 1980, we bought a company that makes Painter caps for large Paint Manufacturers. During the 80's, it was a huge fad to wear painter caps. We once had an order of custom painter caps for the Back Street Boys for one Million painter caps.

We make aprons, Tote bags, Tablecloths, Tee Shirts, and so much more. Our Adcapitol website is www.adcapitol.com.

Now I make phone calls and use emails most of the time. Remember when we had to call and mail quotes and purchase orders before Fax machines and answering machines? I also check several departments to make sure orders are produced correctly and on time. We also make name tape for military tags, and we offer screen printing and Direct Embroidery for caps, aprons, Tee Shirts, painter caps, Tote Bags, and our other 300 products we offer such as our Drop Cloth Sundries under Mutual Drop cloth.

What's something that you did at work that you're proud of?

In the year 1981, I went to Chicago for the National Hardware Show, displaying our Paint Sundries under the name of our company Mutual Drop Cloth Company. I displayed Nail aprons, Waist Aprons, Shop Aprons, Drop cloths, Paint paddles, and Paint strainers.

At approximately 4:45 pm Thursday afternoon- A well-suited man in his 40s came walking up to my booth. He said, "Young man! Do you make inexpensive paper caps? I said, "Yes, I do." Can you give me a good Price Tomorrow? He said I will contact you Friday afternoon for a price. I asked him, "What is the name of your company? He said, “I am starting a new company called “Home Depot” I said, Great! Talk with you soon. I called him Friday and gave him a price of .31 each for our disposable printed caps. He said, “I will get back to you soon with an order.”

He called after a few days with an order of 500 PC-100 Paper painter caps. He called me one week later and said, “Can you make Our Orange Bibb Aprons?” It will be our logo as well. I said, “Yes, We Can! Can you make us a sample to review? He said, “These are the dimensions with the pockets,” and send me your standard Orange Twill with our company logo. We have been making Home Depot Orange Aprons since 1981, and still today… we make them!

Little did we know at the time Home Depot would become a large corporation.

What did your parents do for work?

My Dad worked in his Grandfather's textile business in Philadelphia up to the age of Thirty years old and then moved to Charlotte, NC, in 1959. My Dad opened up the textile factory in Monroe, NC, to expand the business in the south. Monroe, NC, is located about 30 miles east of Charlotte, NC, off of Hwy 7 4.

My grandfather (Dad's father) Herman Dunn wanted to expand our textile company to get lower labor costs, and mostly customers in the Southeast part of the country.

My Dad bought a factory in Monroe, NC. It was an old mill that was used as a cotton gin from 1900; Then used as a Beer brewery in the 40's-till mid 1950s. My Dad bought the mill in 1960, and Monroe Textile was born. We specialize in Bias Binding, Cord edge, and assorted types of trims.

We produce Bias Binding from customer fabric and Bias Binding from our broadcloth in 100 different colors. In 1981, we started making aprons and painter caps. Printed Tee shirts, Tote bags, and so much more (Promotional Products.)

In 1980, my first bias-binding TRIM order was from the shirt maker HIS. It was a Red /White /Blue trim sewn on the collar of ladies' blouses. This was my first business trip to NEW YORK city.

I wanted to be a stock broker after Graduation, however, my father wanted me to try working in the family Textile Company.

My oldest brother Lance came into the family business in 1977, and my Twin brother Steve and I came into the business in 1980. My middle brother Gary came into the family business in 1982. My Brothers Gary and Steve left the business for different reasons. Lance and I continue to work in our family textile company “Dunn Manufacturing” presently.

My father wanted to be a stock broker after going to first-year college in 1947. Dad went to Swarthmore College, part of Penn State at that time.

Penn State wasn’t taking freshmen on campus that year. In the fall, Dad transferred to the main campus of Penn State. He decided to also go into the family textile business that his grandfather started after coming to America in 1900 as an immigrant from Odessa, Russia. He was born in 1880. My great-grandfather Haim Domb (changed his first name to

Harry and last name to Dunn) and wife Bessie at Ellis Island.

Some of my Dad's hobbies were mountain climbing and sailing. Dad was a world traveler who climbed over 20 mountains, some of the locations were Mt. Denali. It is the tallest mountain in Oregon. Dad also climbed Mt. Everest located between Tibet and China. Dad also enjoying sailing at Lake Norman (North of Charlotte, NC) and in the Caribbean.

My Dad also wrote his autobiography published in 2005, "Surviving the Crisis Du Jour," 45 Years of Adventures in the Rag Business by Larry F. Dunn. My Dad worked after college until he died on March 12, 2008, from Cancer at the age of 78.

My Mom was a housewife who raised four boys with the help of Maize. In later years, after us boys had left for college my Mom did volunteer work at the Hospital called Mercy Hospital in Charlotte, NC. My Mom enjoyed doing oil painting and watercolors. She also made stained glass pictures and lamps. At an early age, Mom did needlepoint and petit point pictures. She was very artistic and had a lot of achievements in her lifetime. Mom died on June 1st, 2019, at the age of 88 years old.

Chapter 4
Maize

Mom hired a maid who had answered her AD in the Charlotte paper. Maize accepted the position and she was from Chester, SC, she drove to our home in southeast Charlotte, NC. It was about an hour's drive each way in 1960. She would leave her family and come to work for us during the day. She worked for our family for 44 years. During all the years Maize worked for us, she was more than a maid. She was part of our family even during the years of segregation. Maize helped my mother with cooking and raising four boys through college years and beyond. Maize was at my 5-year Cancer Free Celebration in 1998 and 10-year Cancer Free Celebration in 2003. When she died in 2004, my parents and I went to her funeral in Chester, SC. We sat on the third row, and during the eulogy, one of her daughters spoke about her 2nd family. She said, "Maize loved her 2nd family very much, and she was treated like family."

Maize was like a 2nd Mom to our family. She was appreciated and loved very much! Maize went with us everywhere we traveled too. We did have a lot of looks when she traveled with us.

Our 2nd Mom, Maize, was treated better than some family members. I believe she would not have stayed for 44 years if she did not feel welcome and loved as a family! She is still missed very much to this present day.

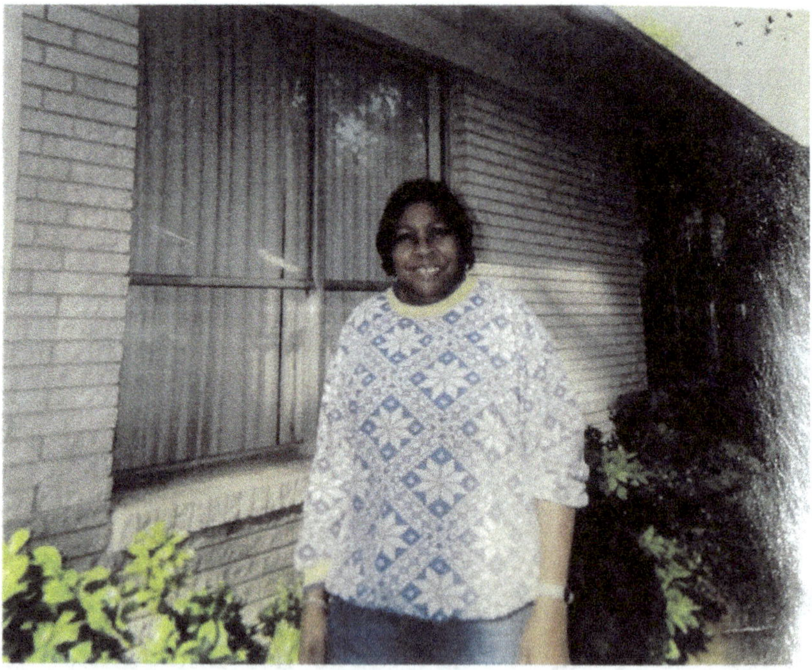

Maize Davis-Our family maid for 44 years in front of Marey and Larry Dunn's House on Lynbrook Dr in Charlotte, NC.

Describe a typical family dinner - who cooked, what did you eat and what were your favorite foods?

Being in a family with four boys, my Mom did most of the cooking. We would normally eat at home Monday-Thursday. We would have Meatloaf on Monday, Veal cutlets on Tuesday, Baked Chicken on Wednesday, and London Broil on Thursday. Friday night, we had the option of eating at home or going out to dinner. I didn't mind eating at home; my Mom was a very good cook, and I always looked forward to dinner.

Sometimes, we would go to some of our favorite restaurants like Dino's Italian Restaurant and Bonanza Family Steak House (The TV show Bonanza started this Restaurant by Hoss, the largest brother with the big cowboy hat). He started a chain of restaurants. The steaks were delicious and had large portions. Other restaurants were Wang Fu Chinese, S & K Cafeteria on Independence Blvd.

On Sunday we would look forward to eating at McDonald's: Hamburgers were 10 cents, Fries and Cokes were 15 cents, and Milkshakes were 35 cents. We ate lunch at McDonald's and had dessert at Krispy

Kreme Donuts which was located at the corner of Hawthrone and Independence. The price was .15 cents each for the glazed donuts. My favorite donut was the vanilla creme filled with chocolate icing on top and a cherry. The price was .25 each for creme filled. The other restaurant we ate at was South 21 on Independence Blvd, across from the Charlotte Coliseum.

Chapter 5
B'nai Mitzvah

(Helps build a relationship with God)

Steve and I had our B'nai Mitzvah twins together at the age of 13 years old in 1970. In its primary meaning, The Hebrew word mitzvah refers to a commandment commanded by God to be performed as a religious duty. In Jewish tradition, a young person begins the journey to adulthood at the age of Thirteen. A Bar or Bat Mitzvah is a son or daughter of the commandment, and as such, he or she realizes that, like a parent, Jewish living provides life, shelter, sustenance, and growth. With every Bar/Bat mitzvah, the congregation welcomes 'our youth to become full spiritual members of the community.

On the Shabbat morning of their Bar/Bat mitzvah, students lead the congregation in prayer, chant from the Torah and Haftorah, and relate the meaning of our sacred texts to our lives today.

Bar/Bat Mitzvah is a great accomplishment that begins with study in preparation, and then in front of the congregation, you have six months of individual study with the Rabbis to prepare for this.

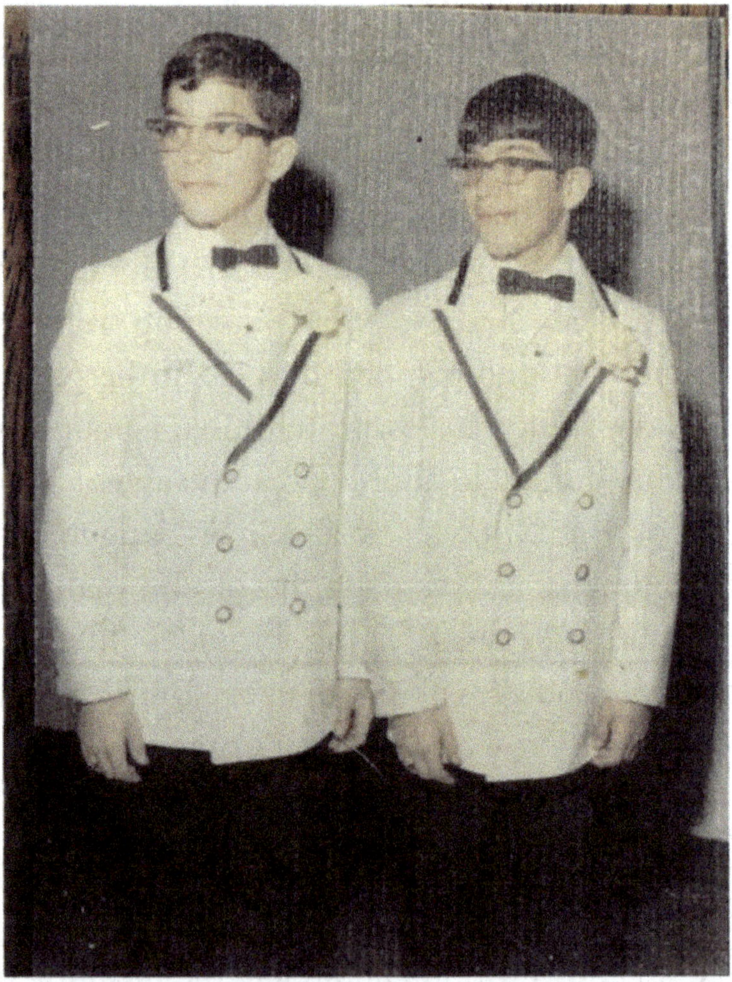

Steven W. Dunn and Barton H. Dunn B'nai Mitzvah
March 28, 1970 13 years old

Chapter 6
Salvation Is On The Way

When I was 23 years old, I was driving near Hawthorne Ave. near the Presbyterian Hospital to Independence Blvd in Charlotte, NC. I drove by an art shop, looked to my left, and saw A picture in the window that caught my attention. It was a famous print in the Bible titled "Christ and the Rich Young Ruler."

As I looked at this picture, I saw myself as the young ruler. I was moved to purchase this picture and think more about my life. I have this picture hanging in the Den, and it reminds me to always strive for salvation and humility. A friend came over to visit me in June of 2013. She also liked this picture, and we thought, "How Cool it would be to see the original Painting at the Riverside Church in New York City." Susan, Dennis, and I decided to fly into New York City early Saturday morning. We left approximately 8:15 am and the arrival time was 9:35 am at JFK International Airport. We had a nice flight, and next we hailed a Taxi cab and proceeded to the Riverside Church.

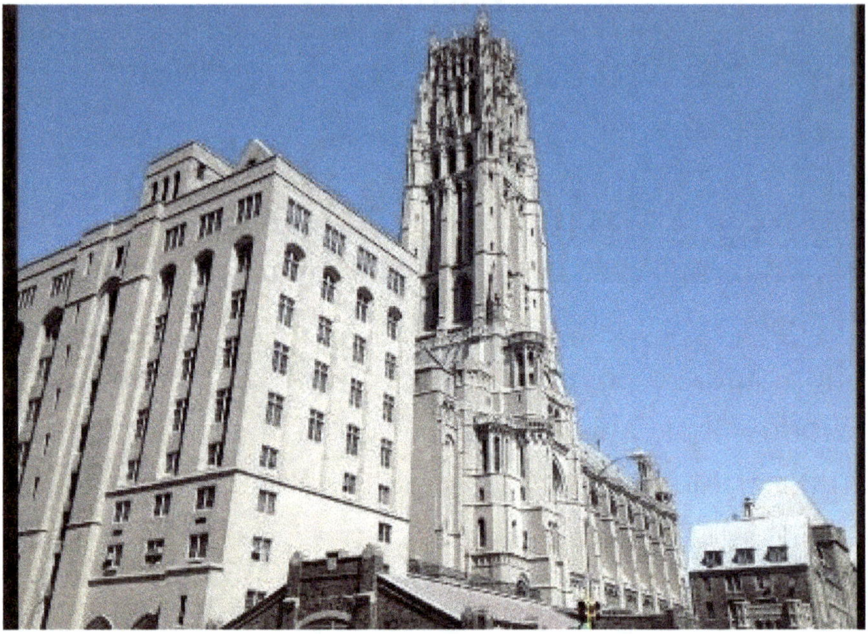

It is located on the Upper West Side, on the edge of the Harlem communities of New York City. The church is modeled after the 13th-century Gothic Cathedral in Chartres, France. Its Gothic tower stands as a beacon to the world and continues to bring people together who have different perspectives. The Mission of the church is to serve God through word and witness and to treat all human beings as responsible stewards of all God's creation. The Riverside church was organized in 1841 and has had three name changes. It was the home Congregation of John D. Rockefeller, Jr and his family. The Rockefeller Brothers Fund was Incorporated in 1930. The Rockefeller Brothers gave personally to build the new church. In the 1940's, the fund's largest combined giving was to the war relief and reconstruction Worldwide. When we arrived at the church, we were ready to view the four oil paintings showing Jesus as the main theme. When I viewed each painting, they were very moving to me. Each Painting came alive with much enthusiasm. We enjoyed seeing the paintings very much.

The paintings were done by Heinrich Hofmann (1824-1911). Three of the paintings were Donated by John D. Rockefeller, JR. (Christ in Gethsemane, Christ and the Rich Young Ruler, Christ in the Temple), The fourth painting, Christ's Image, was a gift from Elise A. Drexler.

The second original canvas, Christ and the Rich-Young Ruler, hangs in the Assembly Hall on the South wall. This picture found its inspiration in the story of the rich young ruler who came to Jesus saying, "What must I do to be saved?" And to whom Jesus replied, "Sell what thou hast and give it to the poor" The canvas shows in a striking manner all of the characters which appear in the story of Jesus and the rich young ruler.

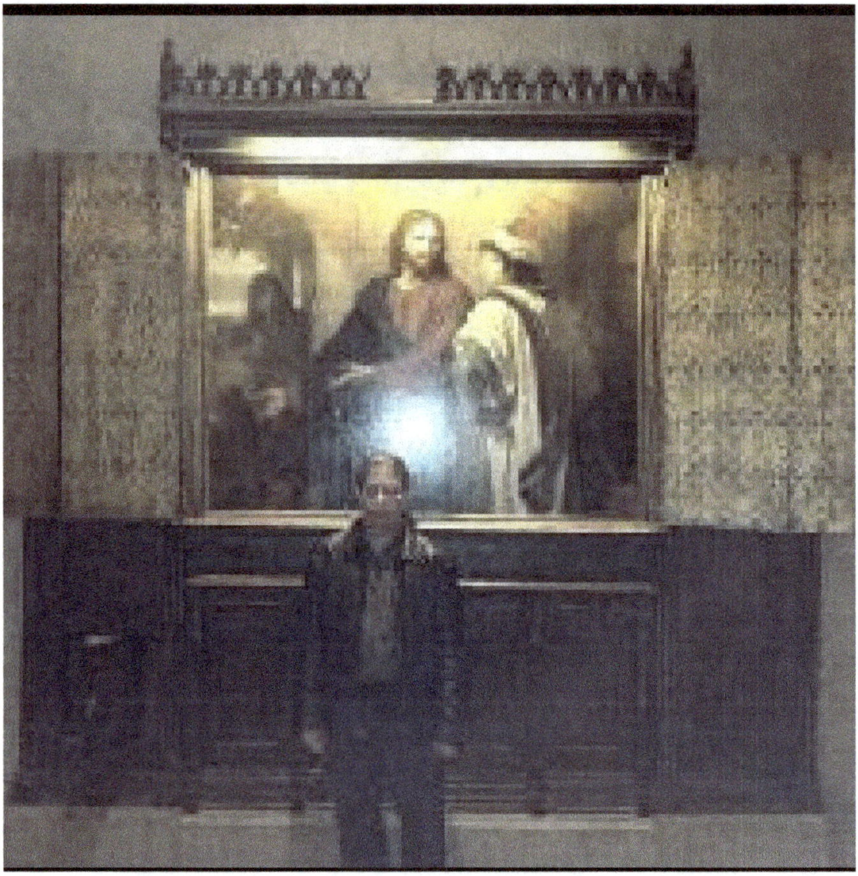

Inside of Riverside Church Assembly Hall

Four are seen in the background, the rich young ruler in the Foreground, sad that the advice that Jesus gave him is not possible for him to follow.

Heinrich Hofmann wrote in 1905, "In my art, it was always of my special interest to represent as Precisely as possible the expression of the face of the human being, in which his soul and his Thoughts are revealed. Only the painting, no other kind of artistic expression, also not the scripture, can reach this goal, and I believe that so many people are attracted by my pictures because of the mental expression that I try to give my characters. Therefore, in the face of the rich young ruler, the shameful turn away from the demeanor of the Lord should be clearly readable-but a much bigger task was the expression in the face of the savior: his eye should go into the soul of the young Man testing him, but at the same time it should express regret and sympathy: for it is written in the Gospel of Mark 10:21 "Jesus, looking at him, loved him." You will judge whether my art has managed This task successfully".

Chapter 7
I Went To See The Doctor

After our trade show in St. Louis Aug. 92, I was feeling like I had the flu so I went to my Doctor in Monroe, NC, and he did some blood work to determine what might be happening to me. The Doctor came into my room and his facial expression did not look optimistic. He said, “Your Lab work does not look normal, SO PLEASE come back tomorrow to discuss this. Oh, by the way, Bring someone with you.” The morning started with thinking about what could be so wrong with me. I had a friend, PAT, who had been diagnosed with cancer the last year in the eight years we were friends. My brain was thinking about all the outcomes of my blood work. Pat wanted to go with me, Pat and I drove to the Doctor's office and went inside. The Doctor motioned me to come inside his office. He said, “Mr. Dunn, I don't have good news for you today. Your lab work shows that your white cell count is very high.

My Shocking Doctor's Visit

The count is abnormally high at 300,000. This means you have stage 4 A.L.L. Leukemia, which is not good. He next said to me, "You should not be alive; that's how sick you are." My response was utter shock and despair. I said to the Doctor, "How does one get Leukemia?" It just happens: one radical white cancer cell multiplies rapidly, and then your body can't fight cancer. I asked the Doctor, "What happens next?" He said, "Which parent do you want to call?" I was in shock and froze and I said, "You can call my mother and let her know."

Pat and I went by ambulance to Presbyterian Hospital in downtown Charlotte. I had passed out before reaching the Hospital ER.

When I woke up, I had been in Intensive care for the past three days. I had a port or shunt in my chest and was already getting chemo in bags and antibiotics. Everyone was standing around my bed (my Mom and Dad, Gary, Lance, Steve, also Pat. I remember Pat bringing in a large vase of Coral Roses (They were put on the nurses' counter). No Flowers Allowed In ICU! I was really scared, but I felt comfortable with my family next to me.

Start Of My Leukemia Treatment

The following day, I met my three doctors at Presbyterian Hospital. 'They talked about our plan of action. First, we get the Leukemia under control and in remission. This includes Chemotherapy, which I would have every day for four months without any breaks. The Chemotherapy took 3 hours, and it went into the shunt in my chest. It lets the chemo go into the main artery so it does not harm the smaller blood veins.

My Mom and Steve would come to the Hospital every day and sit with me. This was always a great comfort and calmed my nerves.

I spent one week in Presbyterian Hospital taking chemo every day; Mom and Steve would come to visit me in the afternoons. Pat was there also for much of the time. Steve felt he needed to be there every day! He would drive 30 miles each way to see me. Steve was so upset when we did meet, so, we talked about being positive and looked ahead for happier days.

This took the focus off the present, and we prayed together every day.

Acute Lymphocytic Leukemia (A.L.L.) is a cancer of the blood and bone marrow. It is the most common childhood Leukemia cancer. It occurs when Bone Marrow cells develop an error in their DNA. I had childhood Leukemia as an adult at 35 years old, and it was around 300,000 white cell count. My Leukemia was considered rare because of these two main factors. The doctors said, “You have to keep your counts in remission because you will die in approximately three months. Your option is to get a Bone Marrow transplant and try to survive.”

How does one know if they might have Leukemia? The symptoms are pain in the bones, whole Body fatigue, High fever, loss of weight, night sweats, bleeding gums, easy bruising, infection, nose bleeds, swollen lymph nodes, and severe headaches. I experienced many of these symptoms, like four months of severe headaches, night sweats, painful joints, and whole-body fatigue.

What is the biggest indicator of Leukemia? Your Doctor will conduct a complete blood count (CBC) to determine if you have Leukemia.

This test may reveal if you have Leukemia cells. Abnormal levels of white blood cells and abnormally low red blood cells or platelet counts can also indicate A.L.L is more likely to cause symptoms that appear over a few weeks. People often feel ill quite quickly. Most symptoms are caused by Leukemia cells filling the bone marrow. After my first two weeks of chemo, my hair was already coming out.

I had Pat cut my hair short, so it was not as dramatic for me. Finally, all the hair on my body came out, including eyebrows, facial hair, and eyelashes. My entire body was as hairless as a Billiard ball. With no hair, you feel so much colder than normal. Taking so much chemo caused me to vomit after each treatment. I became very weak, and my weight fell from 150 lbs down to 118 lbs after the first month of chemo. At this point, neither Pat nor I had the strength to drive our cars for treatments and appointments. My parents hired a driver to pick me up each day and drive to Presbyterian Hospital.

Sometimes, I would have to stay after the Chemo treatment for a blood transfusion. Each Friday, I had a shot of chemo injected into my spinal cord, which was very painful. When I was home, sometimes when Pat was feeling very sick, I was able to take care of him. Much of the time, I was the one feeling sick from all the Chemotherapy. During the time from August to mid-December 1992, I spent time taking care of Pat when I was not getting chemo and blood transfusions at Presbyterian Hospital to keep going. I had to take off from work because I was too sick. I took care of Pat when I felt ok, and Pat would take care of me when I felt Bad. It felt like we were on a carnival ride each week, not knowing what was happening the next week.

My oncologist was located on Randolph Road in Charlotte. I would visit him every week for a checkup on blood work to see how I was doing. On a Friday afternoon, my mother and I went to MC Donald's for lunch. I was wearing a baseball cap, and Mom asked me to remove my cap. I took off the cap I was raised to always remove my hat when entering a building. Everyone was staring at me. I felt so uncomfortable I quickly put my cap on again. We took our lunch to the car and finished eating. Mom and I drove back to the Hospital. I was happy to get some fresh air.

Close To Death

As the months rolled by, Pat was getting worse and so was I. We decided to make our own funeral arrangements. We both rode to Forest Lawn East in Weddington to make plans. We went inside the office and sat down with the director. I told her our situation and she suggested we plan the entire service for both of us. She understood how we were health-wise. We did not know which one of us would die first or when it would happen. We both decided to buy the complete package, which included the casket, service, funeral car, plot, cement vault, and headstone. Pat picked out the only wooden casket. It was very nice and affordable, however, he had a small problem. The center panel on top showed a large Jewish star. Pat was not Jewish and did not wish to offend anybody, so when the time came they would put 12 Red roses on top of the Jewish star.

In the month of December 1992, I was finishing all my chemo treatments, and my platelet count dropped all the way down to 8 points.

My entire chest turned a dark purple. A low platelet count means you are likely to bruise and bleed easily. The Doctor came in to assist the problem, he quickly started treating the shortage of platelets with a platelet transfusion and certain growth factor drugs. I thought that I would die with all the internal bleeding that was occurring. It took almost six bags of platelets and 6 hours to complete the transfusion and get back to normal condition. Pat went to the gift shop and bought a large stuffed rabbit for me. I put the stuffed rabbit next to me in my hospital bed. It seemed like every day was a new adventure.

Bart's Quilt From Pat's Sister

In August 1992, I was diagnosed with Leukemia stage 4. Pat's sister Angie and her husband came over to my house in Waxhaw, NC. to discuss what happens to me next to treat my Leukemia. It's a malignant progress and a disease in which the bone marrow and blood-forming organs produce increased numbers of immature or abnormal leukocytes. These suppress the production of normal blood cells, leading to anemia and other symptoms. Angie made me a quilt that represents "A new life with a new beginning." The quilt shows Noah's ARK with two kinds of animals going toward the ARK: ELEPHANTS, GIRAFFES, FLAMINGOS, HORSES, LIONS, ANTELOPES surrounded by palm trees. There were white doves in the sky with stars and a crescent moon. I had close friends and family members write their best wishes for me on the front side. When I took this quilt to Emory Hospital, I put this on the wall in my room, for inspiration and hope for my doctors, nurses, and visitors to show God was in control of my life. In Romans 8:28, "And we know that for those who love

God, all things work together for good, for those who are according to his purpose." Sometimes, other patients came by my room to say "Hello", the quilt gave patients a boost to their Mental Health. This quilt represented hope and to look forward to better times in the future.

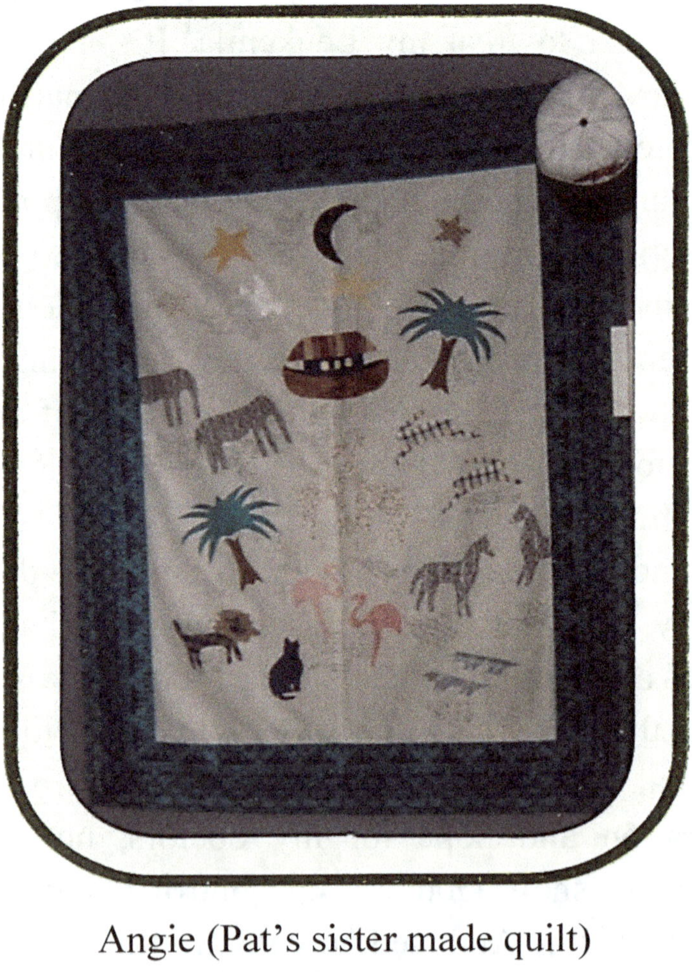

Angie (Pat's sister made quilt)

Chapter 8
Hanukkah Dinner With Family

Although I am Jewish by birth, I am Christian by faith. After feeling better and getting out of the Hospital, it was time with my family to celebrate Hanukkah in Dec 1992. We met at my parents' house in Charlotte, and the entire family showed up. And everyone, including my nieces and nephews, came over to celebrate. Lighting Hanukkah candles, exchanging gifts, Chinese food, and potato Latkes Pancakes. We had a nice time, and after the party was over, Mom and Dad took Pat and I into the den. Mom said, "Bart, Pat- I believe a trip to Disney World would be a great trip for you both to do something fun since you two have gone through so much in the past few months." I agreed, and Mom and Dad arranged everything for a fun-filled trip, including airfare, the Polynesian Hotel, and a 10-day trip pass for two. We were so excited we both cried with Joy for the gift from my parents that would bring some happiness into our lives for a change.

The only other thing to get was a wheelchair; if either one of us was too tired walking, the other could get pushed in the wheelchair.

My doctor said, “I had all the chemo I needed before heading off to Disney World.” We enjoyed all the rides, including the skylift over the different sections of the park. We liked the shows that included rides, and I liked Magic Kingdom. We came back from our trip to Disney World, full of fun and relaxation. We had a great time and enjoyed everything; Just a little tired.

Chapter 9
Emory Hospital
Bone Marrow Match

By the end of January 1993, I was ready for Emory Hospital and the Bone Marrow Transplant.

A Bone Marrow Transplant is a procedure that infuses healthy blood-forming stem cells into your body to replace bone marrow that's not producing enough healthy blood cells. The donor lies face down, and a large needle is put through the skin and into the back of the hip bone. It's pushed through the bone to the center, and the thick liquid bone marrow is pulled out through the needle. This is a very painful procedure that takes about 3 hours. This includes extra time needed for preparation and post-procedure care, especially if you receive intravenous sedation.

My oldest brother Lance checked out a few hospitals that do Bone Marrow Transplants, like Fred Hutchinson Cancer Center in Seattle, WA, Vanderbilt Medical University in Nashville, TN, and Duke

Medical Center in Durham, NC, and then we drove down to Emory Winship Cancer Institute in Atlanta, GA. We decided that Emory Hospital would be the right Hospital for me. Lance and I checked into the Emory Inn Friday night around the corner from the Emory Hospital. Saturday morning, we walked over to the clinic and spoke with a few doctors and discussed possible donor matches, the procedure, and possible outcomes as a result of having a Bone Marrow Transplant. We spent several hours meeting with Doctors and Nurses and matching up the information to consider the possible problems that could happen to me. We went to the transplant patient floor and saw about eight patients. It appeared a little frightful looking at the patients hooked up with several bags of fluid being pumped into them, some with hair and some completely bald. We spoke to a few nurses and asked them questions like, "How many days are you in the large room by yourself after transplant? How much radiation does a patient receive? What is the overall survival rate from the radiation? We spoke with the doctors and decided that Emory would be the one to pick. We started to drive home and we called Mom and Dad and shared our findings with them. I spoke with Pat, and he thought Emory was a good pick as well.

I remember Dr. Hefner sharing with me what happens from start to finish. He told me the survival rate at the time was only a 50/50 chance if everything was perfect. “It's better than 0% if you do nothing,” he said. This was in 1993, and I had A.L.L. Leukemia Stage 4.

On Feb. 1st, 1993, Mom and Dad, Pat, and I drove down to Atlanta, GA, for my orientation and check-in at Emory Hospital. I was feeling a little nervous and excited in anticipation of my new adventure. I had made it through the Chemotherapy in the past four months. Now onward to the Radiation.

The Chemotherapy almost killed me, so I am very Thankful to God for keeping me alive through all of that situation. We arrived Saturday and checked into my room on the 6th floor of the main Hospital. My room was 6G on the left side of the wing. I met with nurses, nurse assistants, and the staff of each department, from Chemo to Radiation. My Mom and Pat stayed at Emory Inn for the 1st month to help me adjust and stay calm. I knew that our journey for full recovery was going to be a long and hard battle to fight. I have always felt that God was in my life at an early age. Remember?

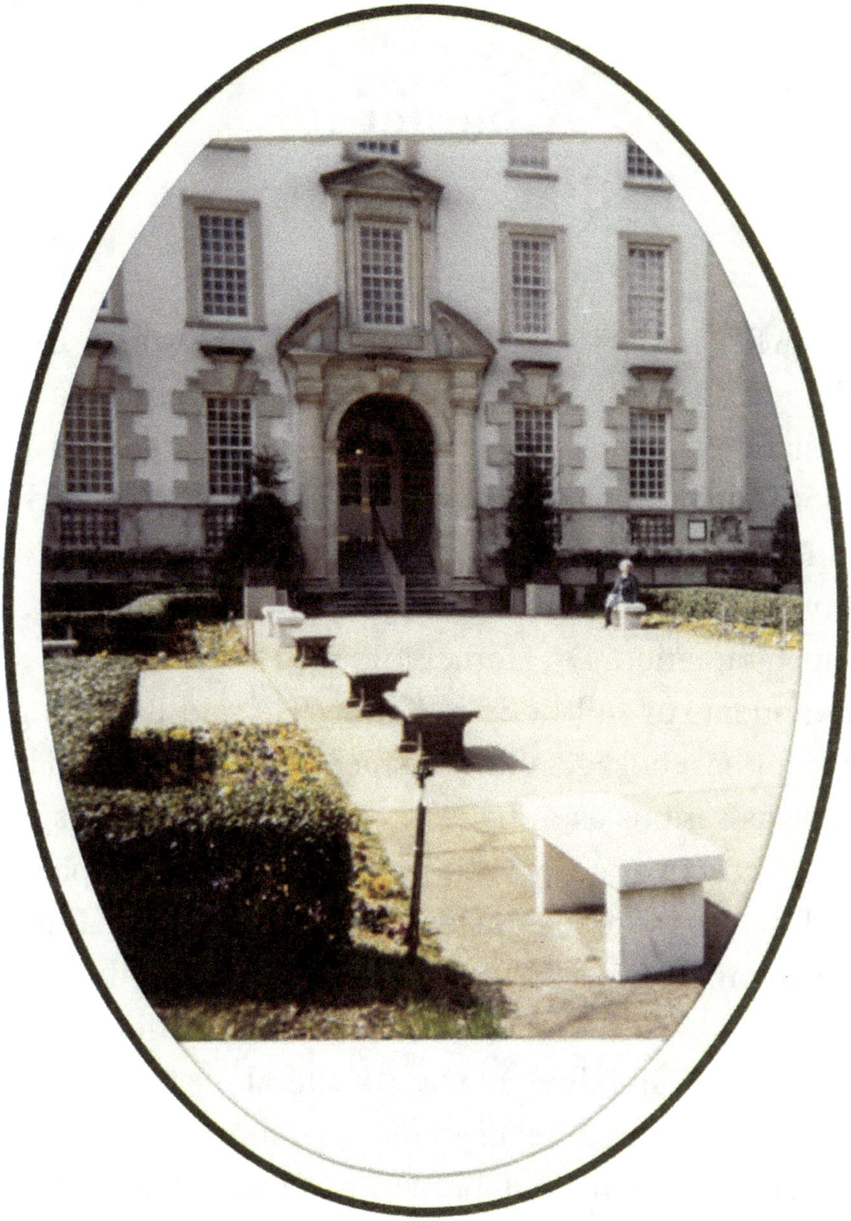

Front entrance door at Emory Hospital – 1993 with my mother (marcy)

Chapter 10: Radiation Treatment

After the first three days at Emory Hospital, I was doing a 24-hour chemo infusion before starting the radiation treatments. I really disliked having to do any more chemo since I almost died from it so much earlier at Presbyterian Hospital. A few days passed, and I told my Mom that I was getting apprehensive about so much radiation. Dr. Hefner told me I would receive ten treatments of full-body radiation. He said I would get the highest dosage allowed since Emory had not had a case as serious as mine. They are a Research Hospital that had never seen stage 4 A.L.L. Leukemia patient before. I would be considered a case study for Emory Hospital. I chose Emory Hospital because the other hospitals also had not a case like mine. I felt Emory was the best-suited place for me. I just wanted to survive through everything. Before starting my radiation treatment, I prayed to God, "Please watch over me and keep me in your hands and protect me." "Amen". On the first day of treatment. The nurse came into the radiation room and asked me to remove my clothes and put this hospital gown on. She said, “Put this lead apron on over your upper chest and down over your private parts.” This was done in order to protect your organs from radiation poisoning and damage to keep your body safe from too much radiation. I felt ok after the 1st day of radiation.

The radiation takes about 30 minutes for each treatment per day for ten days. By the 3rd day of radiation, my body was turning red like a bad sunburn, and I had a fever of around 102 F. My nurse came in and told me that Dr. Hefner would be in shortly to talk with me in a few minutes.

The Doctor came in and told me that my fever would go up by the 5th day of treatment and my skin would look Red like a Coca-Cola can. The fifth day came, and I felt a horrible temperature of 105 degrees F, and my entire body looked just like the Dr. said. The Doctor had my mattress filled with ice-cold water set at 40 degrees F. I was shaking at 40 F and burning up at 105 F, and each day after my treatment made me feel worse than before. “It felt like a living hell.” My burnt skin was crispy, and I looked very bad! I had white lotion put all over my blistered skin.

I looked so bad. I didn't want anyone to take a picture of me. The 10th day came, and my entire body was Red as a coke can, and my body temperature went up to 106.9 F degrees then, I was moved into Intensive Care Unit. I had all kinds of bags hooked up to me and oxygen tubes hooked up to my nose.

My parents were in the room, and Pat and the nurse were sitting in the room, also. My nurse told me she was going to give me a Heavy duty antibiotic. She said it is called Brown Bagging it. Because it was not to be exposed to light. When Barbara, the nurse starting to put the meds into my port. The immediate result was throwing up for 30 minutes and shaking violently for 30 minutes.

I had to endure this procedure for 30 days. This was not something I looked forward to!!

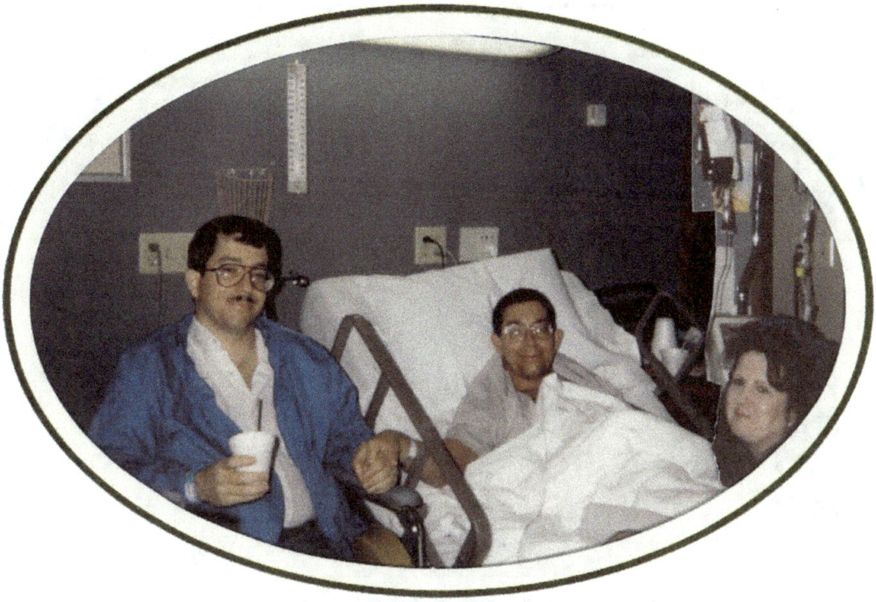

Steve, Bart and Barbara

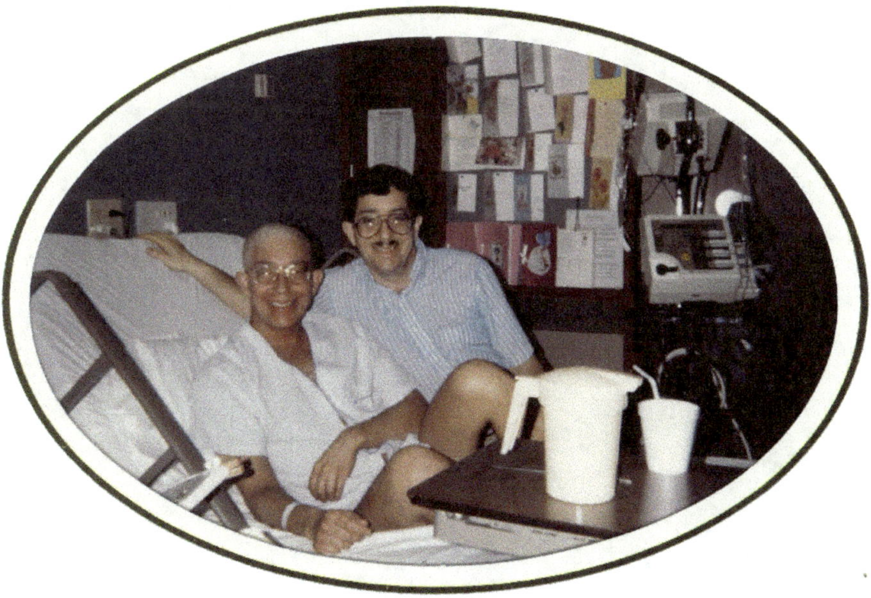

Steve and me

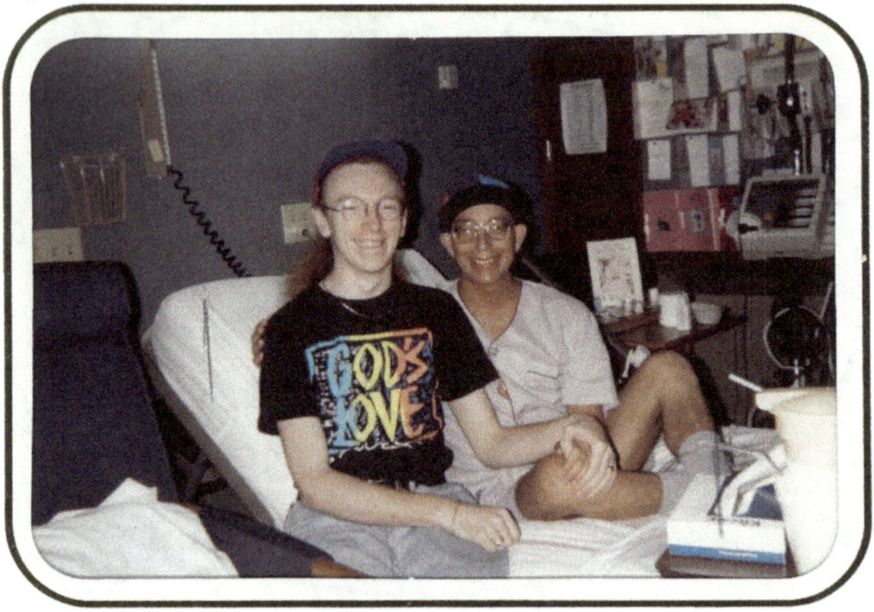

Patrick and me

Chapter 11
Bone Marrow Transplant

The next thing we did was check with my three brothers if they were a match and able to donate Bone Marrow to me. My three brothers were tested, and of course, my identical twin brother Steve was a perfect match! How lucky was I? I said. I called Steve and thanked him for doing this for me. Steve said, "I would be happy to help you, Bart; YOU ARE MY TWIN BROTHER. I WANT YOU AROUND FOR A LONG TIME. I love you very much." "I love you too very much," I said, and thanks for doing this for me.

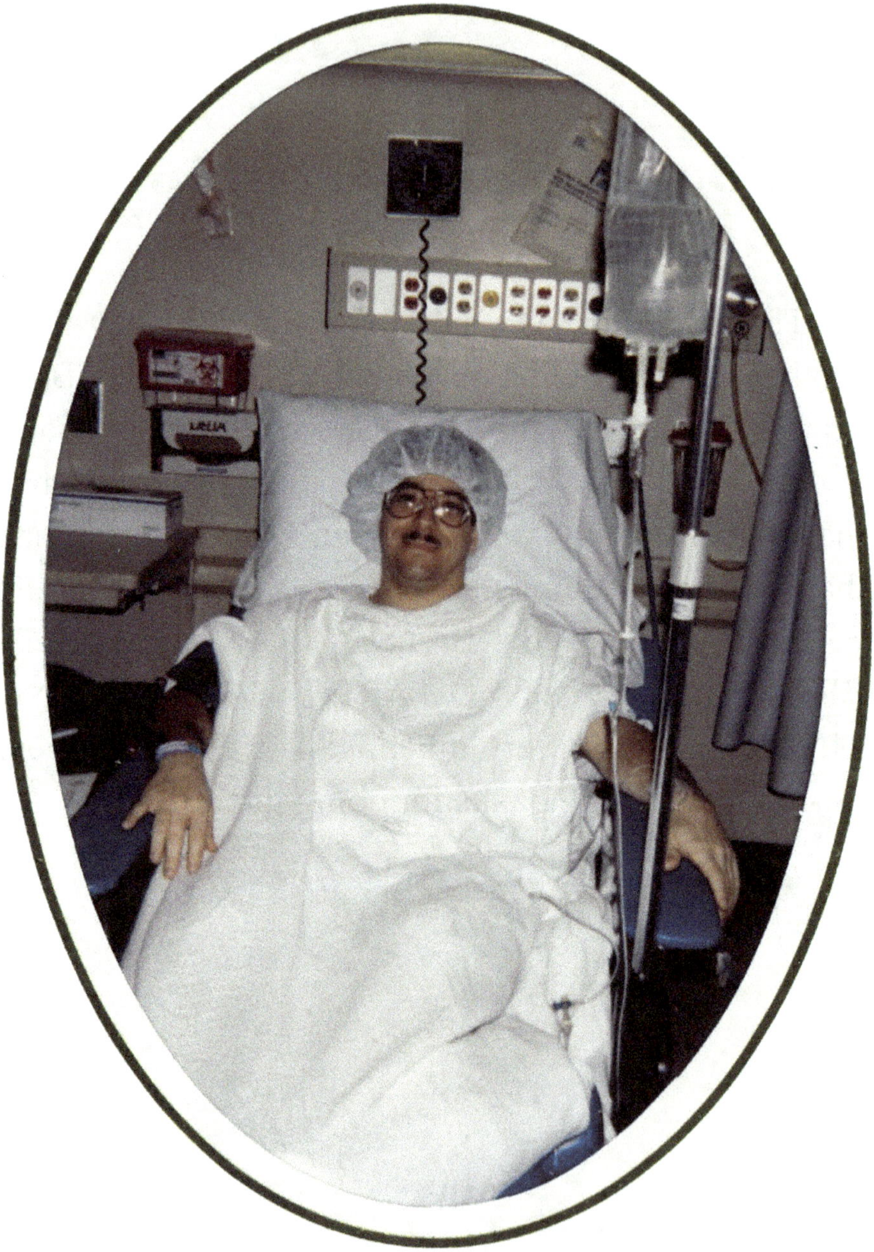

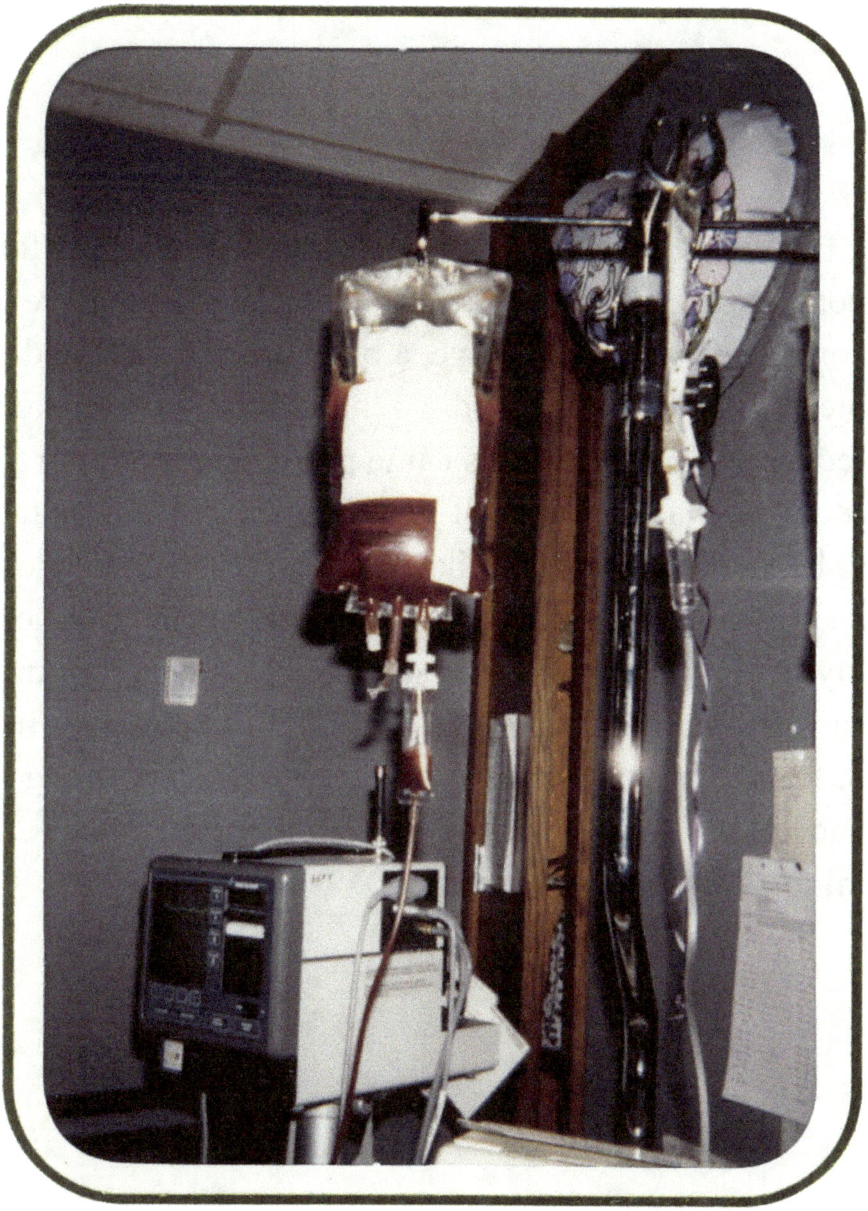

Steve's Bone Marrow going into Bart

I Was Ready To Eat

My Dad asked me, "Is there anything I can get for you?" I sat up in bed and said, "I would love to have a corn Beef Sandwich on rye, a black cherry soda, and a pickle." We all laughed so hard after my spoken request. The other nurses came running to my room to see what was so funny. It just seemed so out of place to be laughing at a time like this. My Dad found a deli nearby around the corner from Emory Hospital. When my Dad returned with the sandwich, I ate everything so fast, and it tasted so good going down! But unfortunately, it was minutes later that everything I had eaten "Just came up." I laid down for about 20 minutes and then sat up again.

Chapter 12
Bart Speaks With God

I had a vision; I looked up at the right side corner of the ceiling and saw "God sitting on the throne, Jesus on the right side of God with clouds all around. I remember pinching myself to decide if I was awake or sleeping! I was awake, and God was talking to me telepathically. Telepathy is communication from one mind to another by extrasensory means.

God was speaking from his mind to mine! We were communicating together. I remember what we spoke about, and God spoke to me, "YOU WILL BE OK, I WILL SPEAK OVER YOU." I Remember God raising his arms and hands over my head. God was speaking in Hebrew, which sounded like a prayer. God spoke over me for several minutes. My Hebrew name is Baruch, which means "Blessed." God said, "You are now healed". I laid back down for about 2 hours, and my temperature dropped to 99 degrees F in that same time period. My red body was fading from Bright Red to a pale pink. I was feeling so well that I rose up from my hospital bed and walked out of my Intensive care room.

Everyone was amazed including my Mom and Dad and the nurses around me. My parents were crying, some clapping their hands, and many other patients and nurses were praising God for this mighty miracle that occurred.

Two nurses spoke to me and said, "That Shekinah Glory" was all around me. It is when a supernatural glowing light appears around a person. This supernatural glowing represents "The Glory of God". I walked down the hall, and everyone was in shock. I walked back to my room, and everything was cleared out. No one expected me to live!

I said loudly, "God just performed a miracle on me. I am still here". I want everything put back in my room like before!

When I was at Emory Hospital in 1993, I would receive hundreds of cards and letters from the local churches in Waxhaw, and Monroe, NC. I always looked forward to opening up my mail.

Most important is everyone's prayers for me. I always felt happy that so many people cared about me. I know it helped me get through the rough times.

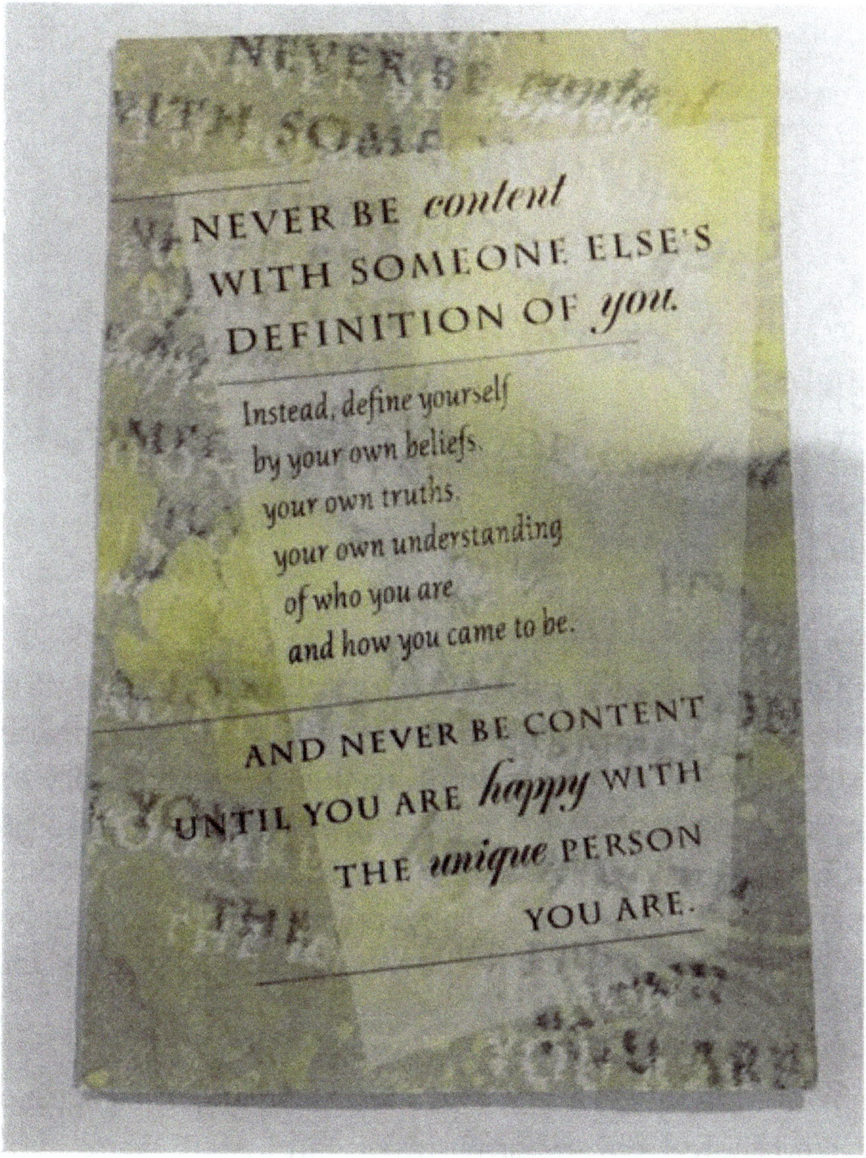

Best Wishes Card

Chapter 13
Shekinah Glory

Ask, Believe, And Receive Miracles!

What is Shekinah Glory?

The Shekinah Glory has happened to me three times in my life. What is the Shekinah Glory? The Bible talks about a supernatural light that glowed around religious objects or in natural Things like clouds. This light represented God's presence. That supernatural glowing light is called "The Glory of God". The word "Shekinah" or "Shekinah Glory" is only found in old scholarly manuscripts. The word "Shekinah" was adopted by scholars as a way of describing God's presence with his people. The phrase "Shekinah Glory" is a symbol referring to that divine presence God promised to Dwell Among his people: "And there I will meet with you, and I will speak with you from above the mercy seat, from between the two Cherubin which are on the ark of the testimony" (Exodus 25:22}: The first time was when I had stage 4

A.L.L. Leukemia, Cancer of the blood and bone marrow when I was diagnosed on August 15, 1992. It happened like this: I had been in ST. Louis, MO. Doing a trade show with my twin brother Steve. "You are on your feet 8 hours a day for five days". When we flew home, I felt like I had the flu. I was tired, rundown, and felt very bad. The first two days, I was very sick after work, and I knew something might be wrong with me.

The word "Shekinah" means "to reside" or "to dwell," with the added emphasis of being a permanent resident in a community. The Bible shows the photo of "Shekinah Glory" of God's dwelling among human beings described as his "Glory."

What does the Bible say about God's glory (The Shekinah)? This was a principal way in which the Lord communicated with his people in Old Testament times.

Showed divine protection and leadership. "And the Lord went before them by day in a pillar of cloud to lead the way, and by night in a pillar of fire to give them light." The fire and the cloud symbolized divine leadership and protection. (Exodus 13:21).

Cloud of God's direction (Numbers 9:15-23, describes how the "Cloud" that represented the presence of God controlled the activities of the Israelite community and assured them on a daily basis that God was with them.

Symbolizing God's presence, this same cloud signified God's presence when the Tabernacle was constructed in the desert: “Then the cloud covered the tabernacle of meeting, and the glory of the Lord filled the tabernacle” (Exodus 40:34).

Located above the ark (Leviticus 16:2) says, “I will appear in a cloud above the mercy seat.” The glory of the lord (the Shekinah) also appeared above the ark of the covenant in the most Holy place in the sanctuary and later in Solomon's temple. What does this Shekinah Glory have to do with me? In a spiritature sense, God's goal.

Chapter 14
Bart Received His Healing

I was very glad to have survived all the poisoning of radiation, and that “God gave me a 2nd chance to live.” And by God and Steve (my twin) I was given another chance to live! 50% of all patients die from the chemo and or radiation before even having the Bone Marrow Transplant at that time. The day after my miracle, my three doctors came to my room (like the three wise men going to Bethlehem).

Each Doctor came to see me separately to discuss the miracle that occurred. All three doctors told me, “They had never seen a miraculous healing.” Like the one I had at Emory Hospital.” 20 years later, I asked if the Hospital would allow me to put a plaque to show the miracle that God had performed on me. They said, “Absolutely, Yes!”

The plaque will bring much encouragement to other patients. The plaque has been on the 6th-floor wall since 2013. This plaque of HOPE AND INSPIRATION over 12 years at Emory Hospital. It is possible to survive leukemia! You have to believe and have faith and always have a positive attitude.

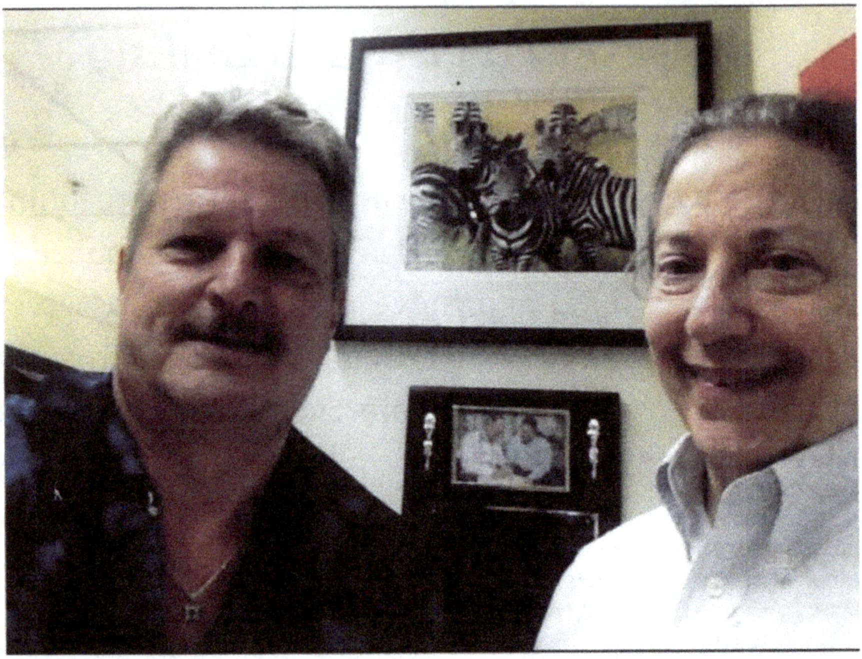

Bart and Dennis with Plaque at Emory Hospital

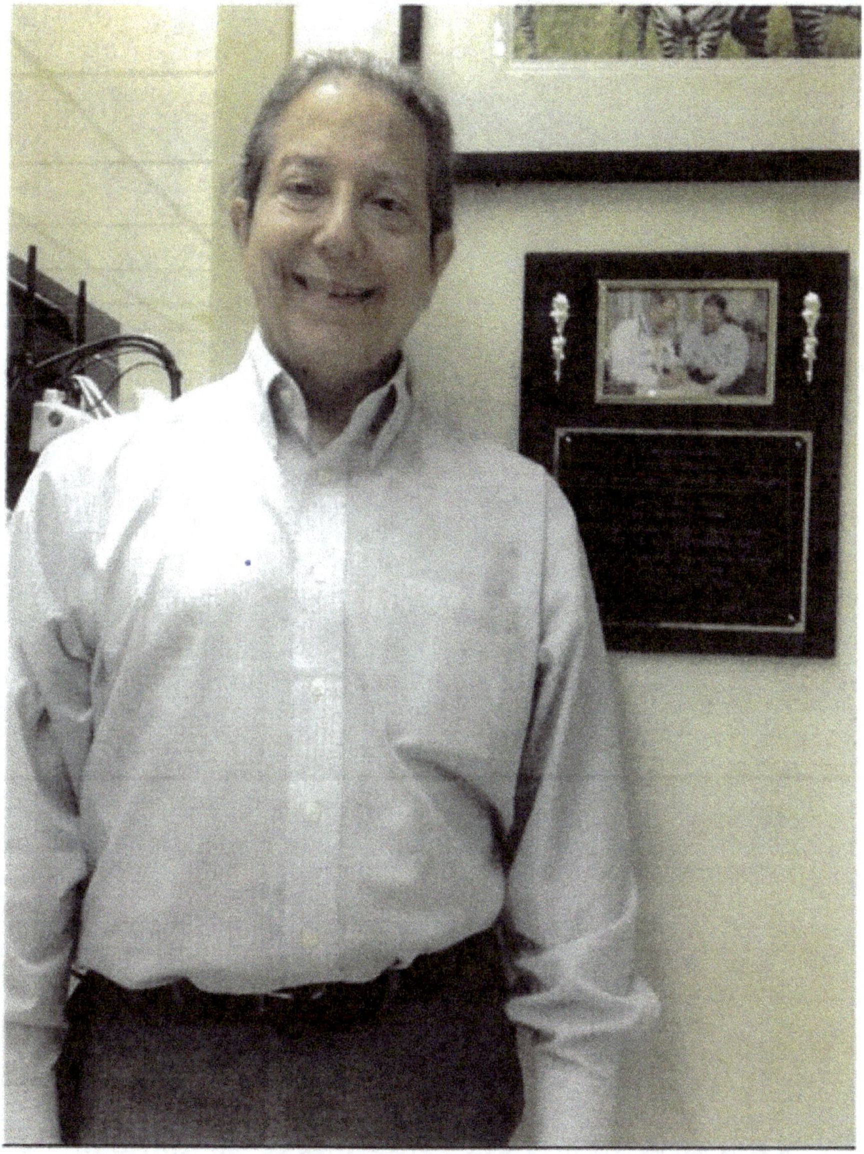

Bart with Emory Plaque

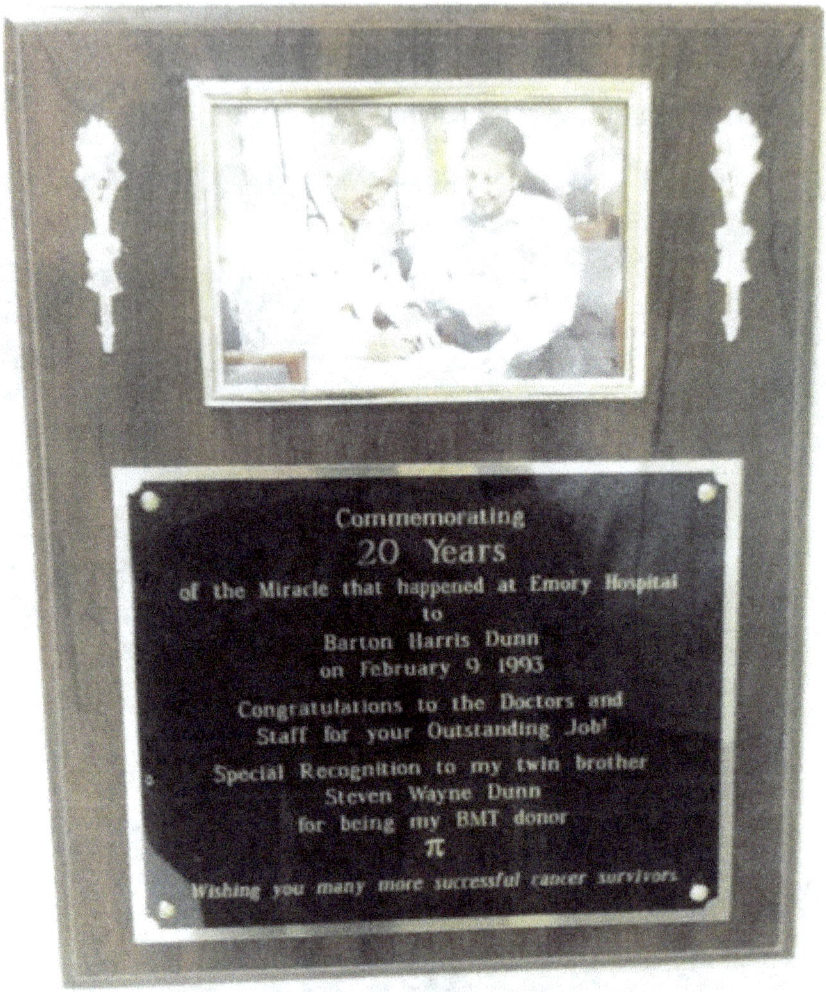
Commemorating
20 Years
of the Miracle that happened at Emory Hospital
to
Barton Harris Dunn
on February 9 1993
Congratulations to the Doctors and
Staff for your Outstanding Job!
Special Recognition to my twin brother
Steven Wayne Dunn
for being my BMT donor
π
Wishing you many more successful cancer survivors

Miracle Plaque at Emory Hospital

I had survived the Chemotherapy, radiation, and bone marrow transplant. I was able to go home on June 3rd, 1993. When PAT and I came home, it was "Wonderful" to have survived one of the most difficult situations in my lifetime. I was getting better each day, and Pat was getting worse each day. Pat's sister would come to visit and help us. It was difficult to cook and clean the house, so friends donated time, and we appreciated everyone who came by to help. Each week, two lady friends would come over and bring food and pray over both of us. This was a true act of love and compassion toward both of us. They were from the local churches in Waxhaw, NC. These two ladies were a great help as the days went by, and Pat's health was getting worse. His treatments were not working for him anymore.

I came to Pat's bedside, held his hands, and gave him permission. He could go to heaven. Pat said to me, "If it's possible, I will send you someone as close like me to take care of you." As Pat became very ill in the last days of his cancer, my parents planned in advance a trip to Israel. On Friday night, they asked Pat if he felt well enough so they could have a week's vacation in Israel. Both of us agreed they should take their trip, and they flew out Saturday morning. While watching TV Saturday night around 9:30 pm, July 3rd, Pat had a serious stroke that left him unable to speak. I was so upset that I called Pat's family to come by the house, and they came over with the Pastor. I had asked Pat's family if they could stay at my home during the weekdays. My Mom called Monday afternoon because she sensed something was wrong. I told Mom what happened to Pat and they cut their trip short and flew back to Charlotte as soon as possible. They arrived on Thursday afternoon and came right to my house. My parents had brought back with them a handmade wooden cross. Mom put that cross in Pat's hands, and tears flowed from Pat's eyes. Pat's health got worse, and he died on July 10, 1993.

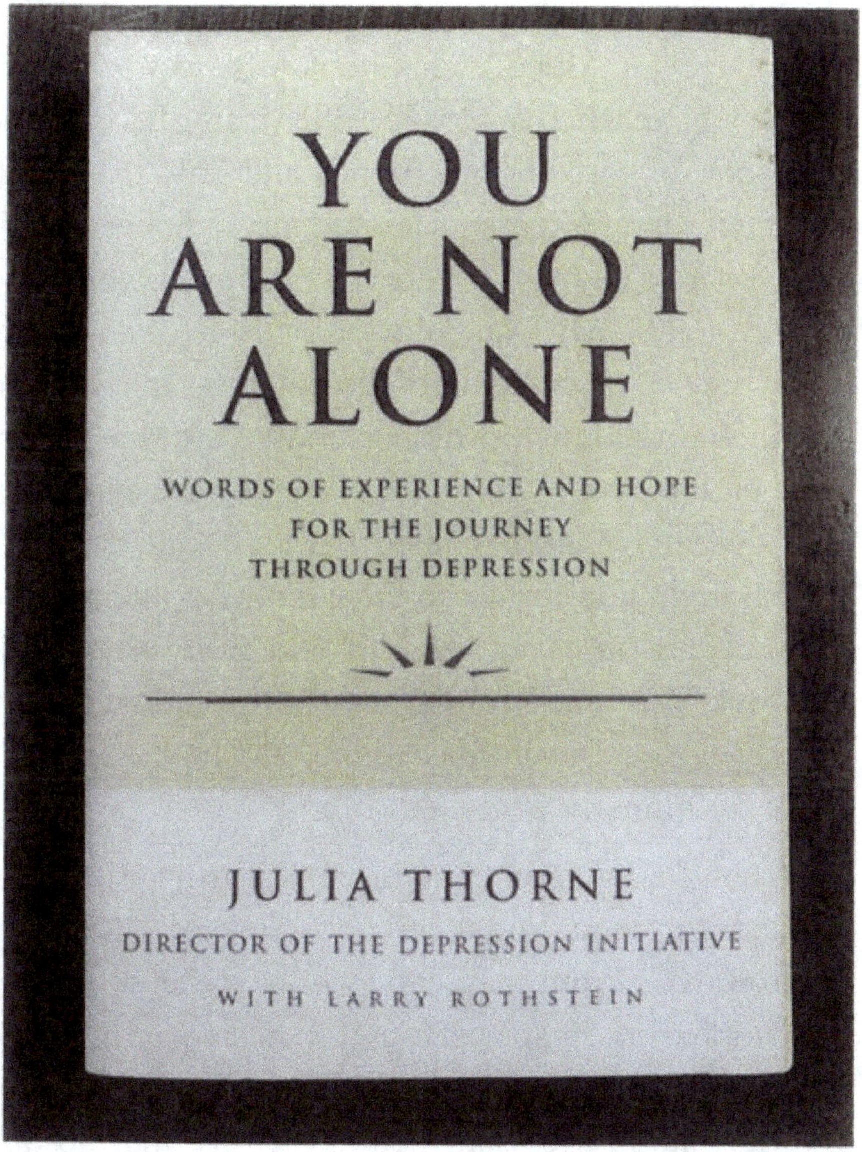

"You are not alone" Book given to me from Mom after Pat's death

After Pat's death, my Mom gave me a book called "You Are Not Alone." This book was an account of people who reached out to God after losing a loved one etc. (spouse, partner, and friend) and how they dealt with their loss. My parents invited me to dinner at their home on a Friday night. I drove up from Waxhaw and arrived at 6:30; My Dad pulled into the driveway at the same time. We came into the kitchen and greeted Mom. We sat down to dinner and a card was at my place on the table. Mom said, "Open up the card from your dad and me." I opened the card, and it was a written invitation for me to have dinner at their house every Friday night for a year. I was grateful for their generous offer, and I said, "Yes, that would be great!" I spent most of my Friday nights at Mom and Dad's house for dinner.

When I survived Leukemia, I was truly Blessed. I decided to be a volunteer for Hospice House in Monroe, NC. From the year 1994 until 2004, when I had worked at Hospice House. It was a remarkable experience sharing my time with others who may not have any family to visit them. I believe that no one should have to die alone. When I shared my Leukemia story, others said to me, "Wish I could take your pain away.

I have two commemorate bricks at the hospice - first house One brick is in memory of Pat's passing the second to celebrate Steven and our 40th birthday together.

I continue to share my testimony each and every day, as God had directed me to do. Make each day count, be happy and have a positive attitude. Miracles won't happen if you don't believe in them.

You will never know where to find them, they may even be put in your pathway. One of the best compliments I have ever received, I once spoke with a young man who had just been diagnosed with leukemia.

He felt like it was too hard to fight the battle. He said, "I can't do this by myself." I convinced him to have the treatments and transplant. I told him that if I can beat cancer, then you can beat it. I first prayed with him and gave him will power to ask God to give him strength. Next, Ask God for daily help and healing. Ask, Believe, and Receive!

I said to this young man, "God loves you, and his son died on the cross for your healing." Ask God to forgive you of all sins. I called John every week and stopped by the Hospital when he had the Transplant.

God healed John, and he is doing well now. Praise God for his Mercy and Grace.

Prayer goes a long way when you are Faithful and believe.

Chapter 15
Trip To Israel

I decided to stop by this church on a Sunday morning for the 11:00 am Service. It was the church up on the hill with the tall bell tower. I went inside and sat on the front row; I felt God's presence all around me. I knew this was the right church to visit.

After the Weddington Church service, the Pastor said," The church is planning a 10-day trip to Israel; you can sign up for that now or later. I leaped to my feet and was the first person to sign up. I had been praying for the opportunity to travel to Israel for a long time. The trip was from May 10- May 20, 1994. I decided that I needed someone for a travel companion for ten days. My health was better, but I still needed help getting around. I placed an ad in the Charlotte paper for "Trip companion need for a 10-day trip to Israel. All expenses paid including plane fare, Hotel, and Food. The first responses were strange, so the 4th person was Tom from Indian Trail, NC.

I met Tom's family and shared some of my health reasons why I needed a companion. They understood my situation, and Tom agreed to go on the trip with me. My own family thought it was crazy to place an ad in the paper but agreed with me that someone should go with me to help.

We arrived in Israel, and we loaded the bus to go to the 7 Arches Hotel in Jerusalem. It was a beautiful Hotel overlooking the city. We traveled to the Sea of Galilee (the largest freshwater lake in Israel). Also called Lake Tiberias. We took an hour-long boat ride and enjoyed this very much.

Some other places were the Valley of Death, where the side of the walls had caves carved out for protection and homes. We went to the Dead Sea too, it was so salty you could float on top of the water. Just make sure you don't get water in your eyes! We went to several church locations and the burial site of Jesus and King David. Our group size from our church was about 25 people, and when we arrived at the Jordan River, only eight people volunteered to be Baptized. All the participants changed into a white cheesecloth robe before entering the water. Tom was in front of me, and then it was my turn.

The water was about 3 feet deep and around 30 feet wide at the point of the baptism. The water was not very cold, it was a very comfortable temperature. The Pastor said to me before entering the water, “Close your eyes and hold your breath as I dunk you under.” He dunked me under, and as I came up out of the water, several people commented about me having a glow all around me. I believe this was the 2nd “Shekinah Glory”. The glowing light around me represents God's' presence, known as “The Glory of God.” A few more church members decided to get Baptized, and afterward, we walked back to the bus and drove to the hotel. It is now toward the end of 10 days. We had seen many sites, and everything looked just like the pictures in the Bible but better in person. We all believed this was One of the most exciting trips of a lifetime! We flew home and talked about the trip, “Next year in Jerusalem”.

This was said at the end of the Passover Prayer, the last supper.

When we arrived back home, Tom said, “Thank You very much for taking me on this trip. I truly appreciate your Kindness and Generosity”. I have spoken to Tom a few times since our trip together. We both learned much while traveling together. I believe that “an act of Kindness goes a long way, Pay it Forward.”

Chapter 16
Was It God?

It is now the future, and the year is 1995 July. I'm at home in Waxhaw, NC, watching TV at about 8:00 pm. All of a sudden, I heard a Loud noise from the master bedroom. It sounded like someone opening up the screen doors from inside and letting them slam shut. This really scared me because Its impossible for those screen doors to open and close when the screen doors are locked from the inside. I was in my house alone, I thought. I then said loudly, "Are you God or a Spirit?" I heard a voice say, "I am that I am." I realized at that moment it had to be God speaking to me. I bowed down with my face to the floor. I started to hear music coming from the master bedroom. I got up and walked to the bedroom, I immediately felt like someone opened up an oven door, and a wave of warm air hit me hard. I heard a lady singing a beautiful song so clearly that I started to hum along with her singing. I felt at peace, relaxed and in no pain. I said, "IF THIS IS HEAVEN, I AM READY TO GO NOW"! The lady stopped singing and I then walked out of the bedroom back to the living room.

I bowed down face to the ground, and I boldly asked God, which I knew that I should not be asking. I decided to ask God my questions, "Why did I get Leukemia? God Answered me, "I allowed this to happen to prove to you that "God is real God is alive, and God still performs miracles every day." While God was speaking, the room was "Glowing all around me again."

This was my 3rd "Shekinah Glory." The light represents God's presence, and that is known as "The Glory of God." I then asked God, "What is your will for my life? God answered, "From this day forward, you are to share your testimony with everyone you meet for the rest of your life." I then replied, "Thank you, Lord, I will fulfill your commandment."

God Speaks To Me Again.

Now, it is Sept. 1995, I had another experience with God. It was early Sunday Morning, around 8:30 am. l was awake and still in bed. God spoke to me and said, "Go to this specific Church in Monroe. You are to visit at the 11:00 am service." That's where my friend Pat and I belonged to, I asked God, "Why am I to visit this church?" God replied, "There is a couple that has lost their son to Cancer. You are to meet them and speak to this couple, and you are to console them and comfort them!" While driving to Monroe, which is a 20-minute ride. I kept asking myself, "What am I going to say to this couple?" God said to me, "I will give you the words when the time is right." I nervously continued to drive until I arrived at 10:50 am. I walked into the church and sat toward the back. God said, "Go to the front row and sit on the far left-end seat." I reluctantly walked down the aisle and sat in the front row. The Pastor was standing at the pulpit and looking around the church, just about ready to start the service. God spoke to me and said, "Walk up to the pulpit and ask the couple to stand up." They were also commanded to go to this church to meet someone like me. I walked up to the pulpit, and the Pastor stood and looked at me and said, "Young Man, why are you up here interfering with my service!" I boldly responded, "God has commanded me to stand up hear and ask if a couple that was sent here to speak with me today." A couple toward the back of the church stood up and said, "We are the couple who were commanded to meet you today." I walked back to the couple and we went into a side room down the hall. I had never met this couple before. However, they were instructed to come to this church and meet someone there today. The lady said, "Wait here; God instructed me to bring a book from home and give it to you." I was very surprised and taken aback by all the events that were happening.

Chapter 17
The Prophet

She walked to her car, brought back a book, and handed it to me. It was titled "The Prophet by Kahlil Gibran." I asked the couple, "Why did God bring you to this church and to meet with me today?" The husband said, "God led us to this church to speak with you today. Our son had died from cancer, and we talked together about their son Michael, who had also died with the same cancer that Pat had died from in July 1993. We spent about 2 hours talking about both Pat and Michael. Our talk together was most comforting to all of us. I thanked them for the book, "The Prophet," and told them to contact me in the future if they wanted to. They said, "Thank you, Bart, for being so kind to us today".

The Prophet book is a collection of 26 prose poetry fables written by the Lebanese-American poet and writer Kahlil Gibran. It was originally published in 1923 by Alfred A. Knopf. It is Gibran's best-known work. The Prophet has been translated into over 100 different languages, making it one of the most translated books in history, as well as one of the bestselling books of all time.

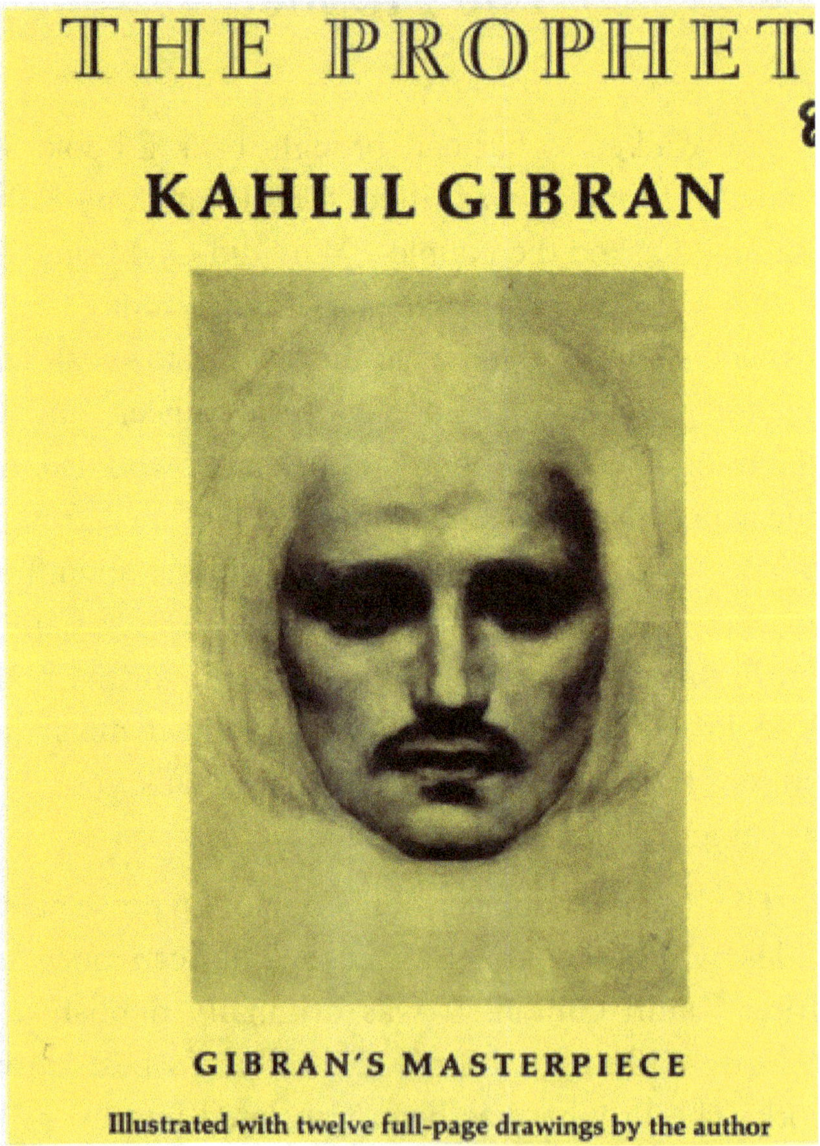

It has never been out of print. The book is divided into chapters dealing with life and the human condition. I still have possession of that book to this day, and I have suggested it to many people that I meet dealing with life-threatening illnesses and cancer.

Chapter 18
Starting My Life All Over Again

I have been living by myself after Pat's death for almost 2 ½ years. I was trying to manage the grief and loneliness of losing my caregiver and friend. God then answered Pat's prayer for me because I had been so lonely. I saw an ad in one of the Charlotte papers that said, "Are you looking for new friends?" I called the number, and a man named Scott answered he had a very friendly voice.

He said, "Anyone who answered the ad was invited to come over to his home on Nov. 7th Saturday of 1995 for a potluck covered dish dinner". He asked what I could bring. I said, "Potato Salad". He said Ok, I will see you at 6'o clock."

When Saturday arrived, I went to the Food Lion grocery store and purchased a tub of Potato Salad, went home, put it into a Blue Dish and covered it up. I arrived at dinner and there were about 20 people already there. Scott said, "Hi, Glad you made it here." He then took my bowl and put it on the buffet table, where there were two other Potato salads as well. I came to this dinner to try to meet some new friends. After talking with several different people, I finished eating and then sat in the living room. A few people were asking a guy with a cowboy hat that I hadn't met yet, "Why he had not taken off his hat?" He said, "He didn't know how they would react," and the guys said, "OH," in a discerning way, they thought he was bald. Then they said, "Take it off, and a few others joined in. Take it off." The man said, ok, but it's not what you think! He took off his hat and, to my surprise as well as all the others. He was not bald but had long hair down to his waist. Everyone was in AW, as well as myself. Then he said, "I told you it wasn't what you thought." As the evening went on, I continued meeting everyone in the room. I saw the guy standing in the hallway who had on the cowboy hat. I went over to introduce myself. He said, "My name is Dennis, nice to meet you, Bart!" He said he was from Grand Rapids, Ml. As we stood in the hallway, we talked for almost 3 hours. By then, most of the guests had already left; we had so much in common to talk about. Both our best friends Pat and his friend Mike had both died of Cancer. We both came from families with four boys, parents married the same year, growing up with the same things in common.

I told Dennis my Leukemia story when we got to the part in my story that Pat would send someone to take care of me. I thought Dennis could be the right one. Then Dennis asked me, "What did I bring for the dinner?" and I said, "I brought the potato salad." Then Dennis asked," Which one? Because there were three different kinds. He said," I brought the one in the blue bowl, and Dennis laughed and replied, "OH, the one from Food Lion?" and I said, "How did you know!" Dennis said, "He has had it before, and if I was going to use a store-bought potato salad. At least you could have doctored it up to taste better, and then I said, "What did you bring?" and he said, "I brought the crab dip and crackers and the London Broil with Bearnaise sauce." At that moment, I knew Pat had sent this man to take care of me because his food was great, and I couldn't cook.

Chapter 19
Our Prayers Are Answered

Dennis told me that in August of 95, he was coming to Charlotte, NC, for a change in his life. He was tired of the snow and cold of Michigan, and, as he was driving down Hwy 77 when he saw the skyline of Charlotte. He prayed to God that this was the first time he left Michigan and was not sure, “Why he was brought to Charlotte, and He didn't want to put restrictions on God.” But prayed, “If he didn't find a purpose for being here by Christmas, he would go back home!” He was living temporarily with a couple he knew from Michigan, Kris and Patrick.

Dennis and I started our lives together after that meeting in 1995 on Nov. 7th at the Pot Luck Dinner. God brought us together, and we felt we had just won the “Jack Pot.” We both received what we each prayed about receiving. Bart receives a caregiver, and Dennis gets a friend. The next day, I asked Dennis to move in with me at my Waxhaw house. It really felt good having a companion and someone who really cared about me.

I have been dealing with symptoms from my BMT, after chemo and radiation. One never knows how the body will react after time has passed from invasive treatments. It causes pain from Neuropathy and extreme tiredness. Dennis and I shared our first Thanksgiving dinner together in Nov 1995 and we took our first Christmas cruise. We planned our trip to the Western Caribbean for seven days. Our first day was in Jamaica, and I had a difficult time walking or standing for a few hours. Dennis had the tour driver take me back to the ship. I was so weak they had to get a wheelchair for me to get on the Ship. We went to the infirmary to find out why I had passed out while getting back on the ship.

Dennis told the Doctor, "I am going to my room to change clothes. Please contact me if you need Too." Dennis opened his cabin door and heard the phone ring." Dennis answered the phone, and The Doctor said, "We are losing your friend." CLICK! Dennis raced to the infirmary and saw Bart lying on the table. My blood pressure was now 40/20. They agreed to give me a shot of Epinephrine to make the heart beat stronger. After the shot, my body was responding back to normal. On Christmas Day, I was back to the infirmary on our cruise ship. I was having some of the same symptoms, so I spent the rest of the cruise in the infirmary. The day before we docked at the Fort Lauderdale port, Dennis spent the day on the beach and did some sightseeing trips since we were not able to visit the island together. The day we got off the ship, I was feeling much better. I felt like much of the trip was wasted in the infirmary. We drove home and saw my oncologist. The following week, I went to my Doctor for a checkup concerning my health while on the Cruise ship. He could not find anything wrong that could have caused that issue.

I almost died another six times from 2 stays in the Hospital with brain encephalitis and three stays with sepsis, full body infection, in the left elbow, and sepsis strep pneumonia.

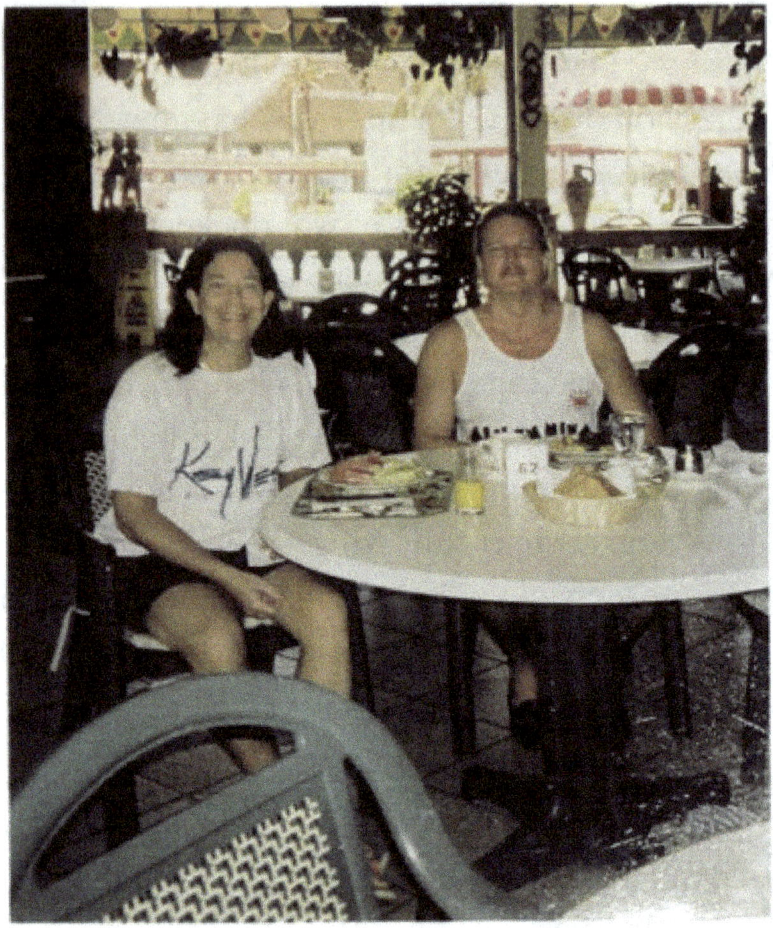

Dennis and I on western Caribbean Cruise

I have been a caring and generous person for as long as I can remember. I guess this was a way of being loyal and putting others first.

We both do our best to help the other person achieve their goals. We have jointly shared many projects to help better ourselves and life together. Our biggest project was when Dennis had the "Swan Manor". This was a wedding venue in Monroe, NC which Dennis owned and operated for 15 years. It was a large Brick Antebellum house with White columns in front. The mansion was 6800 square feet on 26 acres. It was a lot of hard work; however, it was worth having and operating for all the weddings, birthdays, partys and events. Always a positive good feeling time. They have been 14 children born so far that we know of. Dennis sold the house years later in 2021.

We have been together for 29 years in 2024. We have been successful and blessed and have been able to travel the world by land and sea. I know it's important not to put off what you can do today. Be happy and Joyful both in small and large tasks and believe in each day.

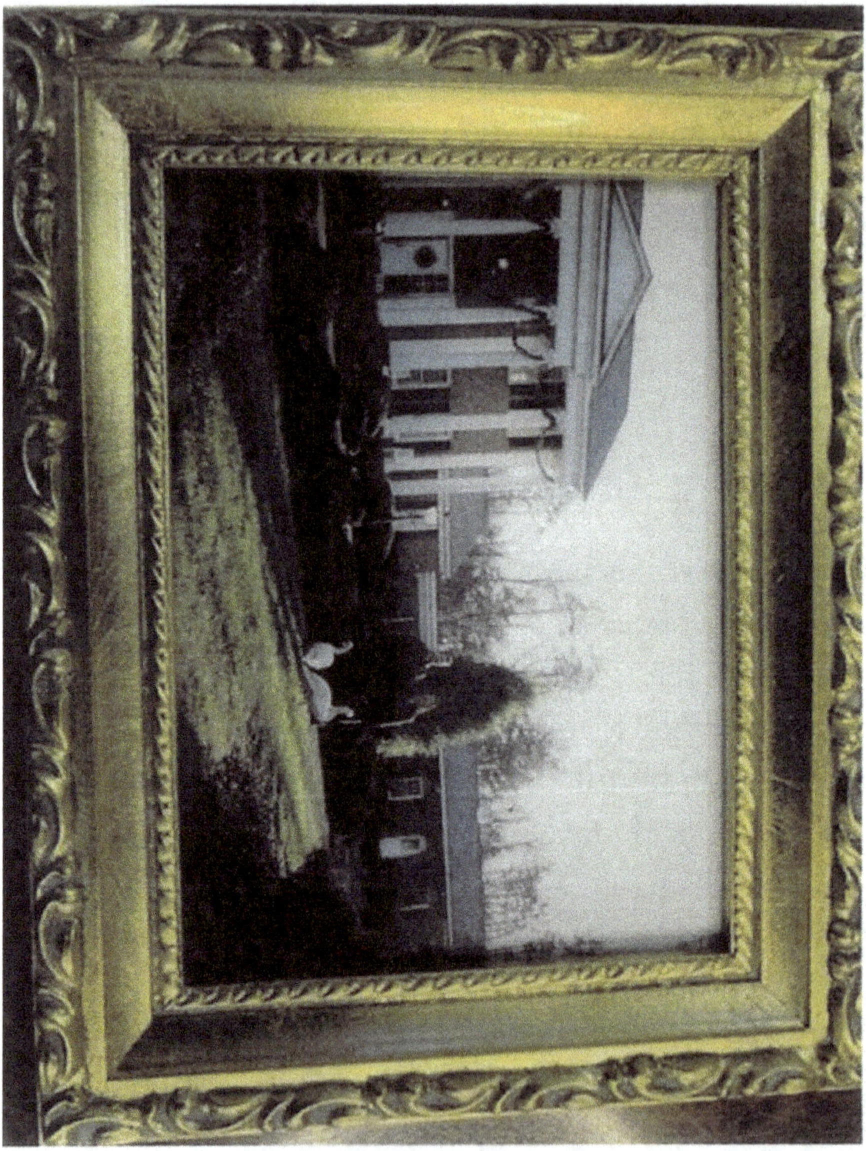

Dennis Cantile – Wedding Venue 2005-2015
(Swan Manor)

Chapter 20
Five Years In Remission Party

Five years after my bone marrow transplant, the patient is considered cured of cancer.

In 1998 (I decided to have a 5-year cancer-free party), Dennis and I had a formal Black Tie party to celebrate the occasion. We decided to have the party at the Henry Hall Wilson house in Monroe, NC. The Henry Hall Wilson house is a beautiful two-story, neo-classical yellow brick home built in the late 1920s. We had about 60 guests in the front three rooms. To the right side was the library, which we used for Dancing with DJ and the far right was the winter porch used as the Bar area. Dennis set up the tables with black tablecloths, and each table had coordinated primary colored napkins and ribbons to match the nametags for each guest. The food was catered with a choice of fillet mignon, chicken, or salmon. We had twice baked potato and asparagus. Before dinner started, our guests could go over to the bar area and get beverages of their choice. The DJ played a delightful array of music.

When dinner was over, the guest had an option to make a toast for me as we waited for dessert. A special cake was made for this celebration. It was a four-layer white cake with raspberry and lemon filling. The icing was white, with the letters in primary colors to match the ribbons, napkins, and balloons. "Happy 5-year Cancer Free". After dessert was finished, the dancing started and I had the first dance with my mother. Everyone took a break after the first 30 minutes and moved toward the front foyer. The foyer was filled with 100 large metallic silver and gold balloons with streamers hanging down. Mom and Dad moved up to the main staircase and called Steven and me up toward the stairs. Mom presented Steve and me with silver kiddush cups with the Hebrew letters L'chayim, which means "To life" in English. These Kiddush cups came from our Bar mitzvah. I then presented my parents with a dedication plague, "Thanking them for all of their love and support throughout my leukemia process over the past five years." Then I gave Steve a bronze trophy cup showing my love and support and for his bone marrow - to mark this milestone in my life.

I thanked everyone for joining me at my 5-year cancer free party. I thanked Dennis for making this celebration excellent, and I love you very much! I thanked Steve for giving me his DNA for my bone marrow transplant and for supporting me all my life. Steve and I are closer together now than ever before the BMT.

I thanked God for giving me a 2nd chance of life.

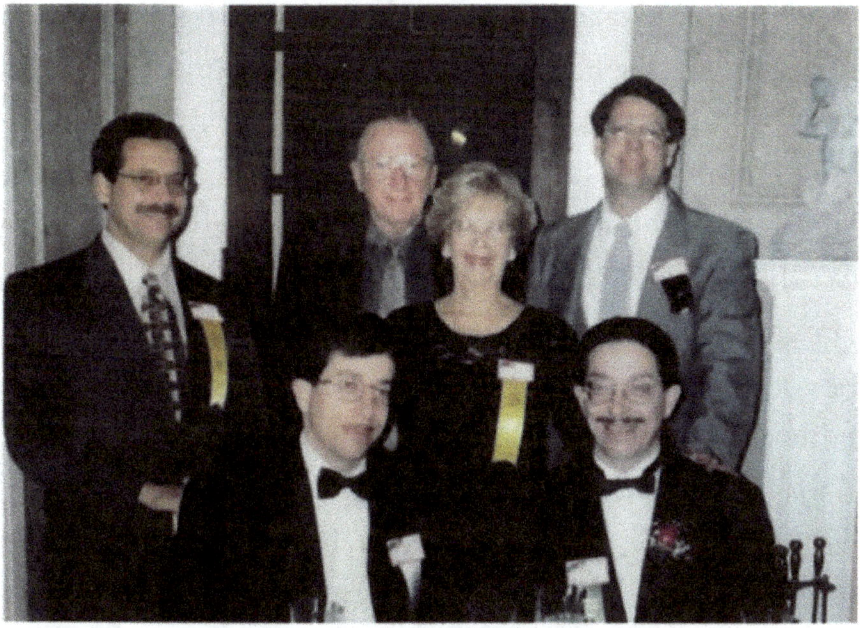

5 Year Cancer Free Party 1998

Lance Dad Mom Gary Steve Bart

Chapter 21
10-Year Cancer-Free Party

The year was 2003, and this milestone reflects a more relaxed party atmosphere. We had about 50 guests at Henry Hall Wilson house in Monroe, NC. We had 44 tiki torchs lining the walkway from the parking lot to the front steps. The attire for the evening was Hawaiian Style outfits. As the guests arrived at the top of the steps, they were greeted with a colorful Hawaiian Lei. and a pina colada or rum runner beverage. The table clothes were white with a square table topper with sea horses brightly colored tropical fish on an Aqua background and sea shells. The centerpiece was round, bowls filled with water and three floating orchids. The front entrance had a large silver punch bowl filled with large shrimp and cocktail sauce. The white chairs had colorful balloons tied to the backside, and we had a DJ who played Hawaiian and songs from the 50s and 60s. We served pineapple, teriyaki chicken, coconut shrimp filet mignon, and coconut fried rice. For dessert we had lime sherbert, with pina colada cake. Some of the guests gave speeches, and some gave me cards. We had a great time at this ten year celebration of cancer free.

Dennis suggested that we bring my quilt that Angie made me of the Arch in Emory Hospital to the party and have all the guests sign the back of it with their well wishes.

Once again, Dennis did a wonderful display with decorations, setting up tables and the food selection. This was a big successful event for all who attended the party. I appreciate everything Dennis does for me, and he does a lot for me! He is truly a kind friend and has been a loving, caring person in my life for 29 years.

Chapter 22
Celebrating 20 Years Cancer Free Party

At Swan Manor this was a country estate that my caregiver Dennis Cantile bought in March 2005 and turned it into a venue for weddings and events. He opened for business in June after the renovations and décor were finished.

On Feb 9th, 2013, I decided to have my 20-year cancer-free party in the Swan Manor ballroom, which was attached to a Swan Manor by a Porte Cochere. The Porte Cochere definition is a covered entranceway to a house or building. They were originally designed as roofed areas large enough for carriages and other wheeled vehicles to park. So passengers could enter or leave the building without being exposed to the weather.

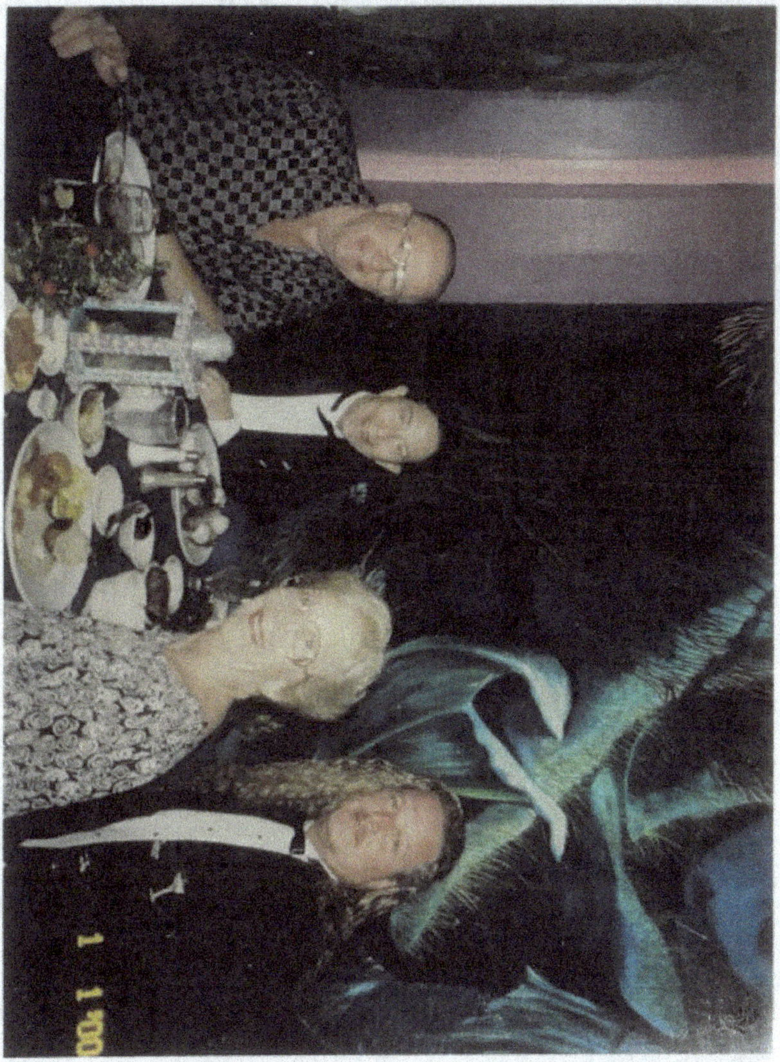

Mom and Dad- 2000 year Aruba Bart and Dennis

The theme for the party was casino night. For my 60th birthday, I decided to buy a slot machine that came out of Las Vegas, NV. I picked out a triple diamond machine that came from the Harrahs Casino and

Hotels in the mid-1980s. The slot machine had been in the Den until it was moved over to Swan Manor for the party. We had 75 guests, and Dennis decorated the ballroom with black and red streamers and balloons. The tablecloths were black with red napkins. We had playing cards and poker chips scattered on the tables. The centerpiece was a silver balloon weight with black and red dice, chips and cards standing up from the centerpiece holder. We had attendants passing out drinks and hors d'oeuvres before dinner was served. Many guests after dinner spoke accolades to me, sharing their stories that meant something special to them. Dinner consisted of pot roast, garlic mashed potatoes and green beans *almondine*. We had a large shrimp cocktail as an appetizer. My brother Steve did something very special for me to commemorate my 20th anniversary. He set up a 100" TV screen and showed childhood and special moments throughout my lifetime, including special family occasions. After 20 minutes, the DVD video was over. I was so moved by the video that I started crying with joy and happiness. After the video, the guests played slot machines and blackjack and had a very nice evening. We had many new friends at this event than my 5th and 10th anniversary. Each milestone anniversary still reminds me how very blessed I am. I love being able to share my testimony as often as possible, almost every day. God is good, God is real he performs miracles every day! Amen.

Had another unique 20th anniversary party in May 2013. This was a complete special surprise to me. In March 2013, I received a phone call from Emory Hospital stating that they wanted to conduct a 20 year checkup on me since having the bone marrow transplant back in 1993. My friend Darlene drove us to Atlanta, Ga. on a Friday night and we stayed at the Emory Inn overnight. Saturday morning at 10:00 am, we drove over to the main Hospital and met with Dr. Tom Hefner (my primary Doctor). We talked awhile and asked "how my health was doing." I said, "I have had a few health issues over the past 20 years. However, I am still here." I went to a room and had some lab work done for an assortment of items checked. Dr. Hefner came back to my room after 20 minutes and said, "Bart, please follow me so I can show you your lab results." We walked down a long hall and came upon a closed door on the left side. I opened the door, and the room was literally filled with nurses, doctors and staff who shouted, "SURPRISE!" they all showed up to see me 20 years after my bone marrow transplant. I was so overwhelmed and delighted to see most of the same staff from 20 years earlier. We had a large sheet cake that had white icing with light blue roses. The top said, “Happy 20th anniversary, Bart”. I was beaming with happiness and surprise. We also had vanilla ice cream and a lot of blue and white balloons tied to all of the chairs. That day, a photographer was taking photos of Dr. Hefner and I. one photo was put on the plague that hangs on the 6G floor wall where it shows the miracle I had at Emory Hospital. The other photos were put in Emory Magazine, which is published six times each year. They had a very good write-up of me in their magazine.

I had the utmost respect for the doctors, nurses and staff at Emory Hospital. They gave me the best care, respect and, most of all, “GENUINE COMPASSION”.

Chapter 23
Celebrating 30 Years Cancer Free Party

On Feb 9, 2023, I celebrated my 30th anniversary cancer free party. I decided to have my party at the Belk Mansion (Built 1903), Right down the street from our Monroe House (Dr. John Blair Home). Our house is a three story Victorian with a slate Roof Built era 1902. I decided to have a disco 70's theme, including an open Bar disco mirrored Ball and lots of colored balloons with hanging streamers. We had 40 guests, and everyone had their best '70s disco Attire on, including satin shirts, polyester bell bottom pants and James brown gangster hats. As you open the front door at the Belk mansion, there is a large crystal candelier. This two story home has three sides, wrap around front porches on both stories. It has four huge majestic antebellum columns on each side of the front door. To the right was the dance floor, and to the left are two large rooms for dining. The round, inlay wood table in the foyer had a large crystal punch bowl filled with once again with large shrimp cocktail. My favorite. The other table had an assessment of cheese, crackers and assorted types of light appetizers. The tables had white linen tablecloths with disco theme decorations on the table; the center piece were vases with GROOVY multi colored assorted Daisies. Dinner consisted of Roast Beef, Grilled Chicken, Garlic Mashed Potatoes and Glazed Carrots with a Dessert Extravaganza! Everything from Banana Stuffed Strawberries to Keylime cake rolls. This was a very nice and high-energy party! I look forward to the next celebration!

Chapter 24
Big Questions

Why do I have long hair today?

When I started taking Chemotherapy on Sep 7^{th,} 1992, for my Leukemia, my hair came out over a period of 3 weeks. I was having my Chemotherapy at Presbyterian Hospital (Downtown) Charlotte, NC. My chemo treatments were five days a week, and the last treatment was at the end of December 1992. I had medium-length black hair, and it all fell out. It was a real shock to see myself with no hair.

The 2nd time I lost my hair was at Emory Hospital on Feb 7th, 1993, in Atlanta, Ga. I was taking full body radiation for ten days for 30 minutes each treatment. The radiation treatment was worse than the Chemotherapy. It took about 4-6 months because my hair started growing back in this photo of Bart after five years, from 1993-1998, with a ponytail about 7 inches long. I look just as good now as before having leukemia. My hair is still black without any gray hair showing.

I almost died from the Chemotherapy and almost died from the radiation treatments. I survived both treatments, and God blessed me with a "miracle of life." Even 30 years later, my hair is still long but now turning gray.

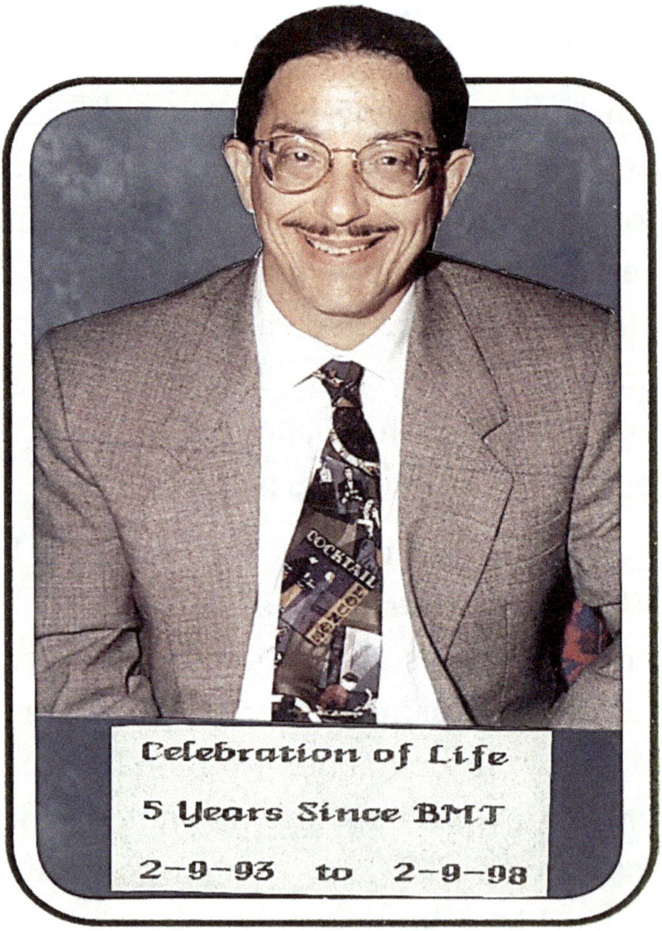
Celebration of Life
5 Years Since BMT
2-9-93 to 2-9-98

My Favorites

Time of day: I like the time after work between 5:30 pm and bedtime 11:00 pm.

Season: I like springtime because it represents new beginnings and opportunities.

Way to relax: My favorite way to relax is walking on the beach.

Author: I don't have a favorite author! Usually read magazines, newsletters and other publications. It's hard to just sit down and start reading a book. It's difficult to keep focused on one story for a long period of time for me.

Artist: My favorite artists would be from the old masters: Rubens, Flemming, Rembrant, Albrect Durer, to name a few.

Musician: I enjoy Big Band, disco music, and Louis Armstrong comes to focus.

Famous person: Diana Ross- I have always liked her music from the age of 8 years old. In 2020, we drove to an outdoor venue west of Washington D.C..

This was one thing on my bucket list – we didn't want to miss!

Movie: My favorite movie is It's a Wonderful Life, "A Christmas classic."

Book: I like the books "The Giving Tree" and "The Prophet."

Animal: Any type of cat- From Household to large Game Cats.

Holiday destination: My favorite vacation spots are Aruba, part of the three A.B.C. islands Italy, and Spain. Vienna, Austria.

Cuisine: Italian and Chinese Food

Restaurant: Landmark Diner Restaurant- Charlotte, NC, Ruth Chris Steakhouse – Southpark (Charlotte, N.C.)

Type of exercise: Walking is my best form of exercise.

Country: USA is simply the best country in the world.

Smell: My favorite flower smell is "Gardenia."

Word: My favorite word is "Grateful."

Quote: "Make every day count," my quote.

What's one memory from your childhood that makes you smile?

In 1973 (I was 16 years old), my entire family went on a vacation through Central America for a total of 15 days. My parents, three brothers, and I started out by car from Charlotte, NC. We took the southern route, going through SC, GA, AL, LA, MS, Texas, and Northern Mexico. My Dad rented a large Gold New Yorker big enough for the trip and souvenirs.

I remember one evening while in Mexico, we were driving down a big hill dimly lit only by the full moon. We were halfway down the hill, and suddenly, a huge cow walked in front of the car and Dad stomped on the brakes, but to no avail. We hit the cow, going about 45 mph. Everyone in the car yelled, and the next moment, we looked in Horror as the cow turned over on its back and slid about 20 feet.

Dad looked behind after stopping the car abruptly to see if the cow was still alive. Dad pulled off the road and walked up to the cow. The cow rolled over and stood up on all four legs. Dad saw a small crowd of locals who had witnessed what just happened. Dad offered the owner a few pesos to show his gratitude that the cow still lives. The next few days, we made it into Nicaragua. We stopped at a small cafe for gas and something to drink. The server said, “You have to watch for the dangerous guerrillas.” My Mom then said, “You mean the little Monkeys.” We all listened as the server explained to us the counterrevolutionary guerrilla campaign by the US-backed Contras. Our next stop was at the Panama Canal. We watched the locks fill up with water and then empty. As the ships came in one end and out the other side.

This is an interesting account of one of the family trips together!

If you could share a meal with anyone in the world, who would it be and why?

I would like to share a meal with Pres. Jimmy Carter who is now 100 years old. At the same time, I was in the Hospital at Emory in Atlanta in 1993, for my BMT Ron, my orderly told me that President and Mrs Carter were on the 9th floor. Rosalyn Carter was having surgery and would be here for five days. I took an elevator to the 9th floor and dropped off a handwritten note to secret service, to my surprise. The secret service would not let me off when the doors were opened. As I said earlier, “The rest of my story.” And she wrote me back a letter, “wishing me a speedy recovery." Mrs. Carter said Jimmy did not have time to visit with you; maybe another time!

I believe Pres. Carter has done more as a citizen starting "Habitat for Humanity."

What advice would you give to your 18-year-old self?

Live each day to the fullest. Make each day count, and be kind to others. I would probably take more risks and spend more time traveling with friends. For every action we take, there is a reaction.

Take a chance; what's the worst that could happen if the outcome is a little different than you expect?

Sometimes, you lose more if you don't try something you believe in, most of the time, the outcome will turn out better than you expect.

What's the nicest thing a friend has ever done for you?

My friend and caregiver Dennis brought me an E550 Mercedes convertible for my 65th birthday.

The color is olive tree gray, and the interior color is dove grey with a black rooftop. It is a sharp car. I get lots of compliments on it.

What's one quality you think is important in a friend?

The number one quality in a friend is Loyalty. The other quality in a friend is, "Trust."

Aside from your closest friend, who else was/is an influential person in your life?

My identical twin brother Steve Dunn. He has always been my closest friend, and we talk almost every day. Steve is the one who gave me his bone marrow for my Bone Marrow Transplant in 1993. We are very close since I have Steve's DNA. Dennis cantile – he looks out for me and does a lot for me as a caregiver.

Anything else you'd like to add about your friendships?

My friendships are long lasting because having friends is important and a gift from God.

How do you define a "good" or "successful" life?

Success is a word that has many definitions. Often, people equate success with money. The fact is that there are millions of affluent "failures" and an equal number of "successes" who have nothing in the bank.

One definition of success is To win the respect of intelligent people and the affection of little children, to earn the approval of honest critics, and to endure the betrayal of false friends.

To appreciate beauty, to find the best in others, to leave the world a little bit better by helping a person in need, respecting the poor and the elderly, and forgiving someone who has hurt you.

To have played and lived with enthusiasm and seeing with exultation, to know that even one life has breathed easier because you have lived.

This is to have succeeded. Making a positive difference in someone's life.

To help another person in need.

How do you feel about getting older?

Live Gracefully. Have style and be a loving person.

How will you be remembered? Set a great example for others!

If we are Blessed and try to live a Righteous life each day, then getting older will be a great life.

I look forward to getting older and sharing my life's testimonial each day!

Look for the love, beauty, and kindness around you.

I believe when we are blessed, we should search out and bless others.

An act of kindness is like throwing a rock into the lake and watching the ripples expand outward.

You never know how many lives you have touched with one simple act of kindness!

Like the phrase "Paying it forward."

What's the best and worst advice you've ever been given?

The best advice given to me is to be an original person, and the worst is to imitate others.

The imitation of others is the greatest form of flattery for them; however, I believe in being an original, not a copy.

What's the best compliment you've ever received?

You have changed my life for the better. You have made a positive impact on my life!

You have shown me compassion, like the compassion of Jesus Christ.

THE END FOR NOW!

You can buy my book online:

1st choice:

* amazon.com(books) under:

Barton H. Dunn "one life to live" – my journey through health, healing and faith, stage 4 surviving cancer.

* Walmart.com

* Target.com

* Barnes & Noble.com

* Books a million.com

If you enjoyed reading my book, tell your friends.

Have faith and Believe in miracles. They do still happen. "Watch for them."

About The Author

www.ingramcontent.com/pod-product-compliance
Lightning Source LLC
LaVergne TN
LVHW022101200926
848481LV00003B/1023
9798348592851